Social Indicators Research Series

Volume 91

This series provides a public forum for authored and edited volumes on social indicators research. It is a companion series to the journal Social Indicators Research. The book series deals with problems associated with the quality of life from a broad perspective. It welcomes research on a wide range of substantive areas, including health, crime, housing, education, family life, leisure activities, transportation, mobility, economics, work, religion and environmental issues. The topics represented in this series cover and involve a variety of segmentations, such as social groups, spatial and temporal coordinates, population composition, and life domains. The series presents empirical, philosophical and methodological studies that cover the entire spectrum of society and are devoted to giving evidence through indicators. It considers indicators in their different typologies, and gives special attention to indicators that are able to meet the need of understanding social realities and phenomena that are increasingly more complex, interrelated, interacted and dynamic. In addition, it presents studies aimed at defining new approaches in constructing indicators. An international review board for this series ensures the high quality of the series as a whole.

Available at 25% discount for International Society for Quality-of-Life Studies (ISQOLS).

Paolo Corvo • Ilaria Riccioni
Editors

Theatre and Quality of Life

Structures, Practices, Actors

Springer

Editors
Paolo Corvo
University of Gastronomic Sciences
Bra-Pollenzo, CN, Italy

Ilaria Riccioni
Free University of Bozen-Bolzano
Bolzano, Italy

ISSN 1387-6570 ISSN 2215-0099 (electronic)
Social Indicators Research Series
ISBN 978-3-032-09730-9 ISBN 978-3-032-09731-6 (eBook)
https://doi.org/10.1007/978-3-032-09731-6

This Springer imprint is published by the registered company Springer Nature Switzerland AG
The registered company address is: Gewerbestrasse 11, 6330 Cham, Switzerland

Introduction

This book constitutes a series of reflections on the potential impact of theatre on everyday life and well-being, with reference to contemporary digital and global society. As a live event, performance holds qualities of a past society, where the idea of virtuality was far off, and indeed also contains some essential timeless qualities for human life and recognition of alterity. Theatre is a powerful and radical manifestation of the relationship between creativity and society.

Through the theatrical experience, spectators form a collective body that resonates in unison, incorporating the emotional and affective dimensions of shared social values.

These qualities are particularly pertinent in the digital era, as virtual relationships are becoming increasingly prevalent in the social construction of society. In today's interconnected digital society, theatre continues to fulfil its role thanks to its status as a dynamic live art form that recreates the experience and the advantages of being present.

Theatre gives us what Greek tragedy did: moments of truth. It confronts us with situations on stage that aren't real, but which mirror fundamental human experiences. In addition, as is the case in Greek tragedy, once the theatrical drama has reached its conclusion, catharsis ensues. This term refers to the purification that rewards the suffering experienced in tragedy, and this is possible only in the context of theatre or in the context of the collective effervescence that Durkheim recognized in religious events, and also today in music concerts and sports events. It is evident that theatre is inherently constrained by its physical nature and the limitations of human interaction. However, it possesses a profound depth that resonates with human emotionality. The spectator is increasingly involved in constructing the collective meaning of the event and is transformed through this first-hand experience—a key element that distinguishes theatre from other arts. In social terms, the impact of theatrical action can therefore be divided into various aspects: theatre as a builder of the public sphere through a political reappropriation of social space; theatre as a means of fostering prosocial behaviour and collective well-being; theatre as a means of pedagogy and socialization to foster prosocial behaviour among new generations; a creative space for expressing the imagination; poetic theatre recovering the symbolic sphere of social life, theatre as a cultural centre for towns and cities; the beating heart of urban communities.

The chapter authored by Ilaria Riccioni seeks to explore the potential of artistic institutions to foster societal well-being on the basis of research on 'Theatre and Public Sphere' (Riccioni 2020). Indeed, all artistic phenomena serve to mediate the socio-political transformations that are occurring in the contemporary global context, as they represent a societal form of self-reflection. In contemporary times, an increasing number of individual actions are becoming collectively disjointed yet are united by the same imagery. These actions are 'affectively oriented', oscillating between politics and society and increasingly reliant on imaginary communities defined by social platforms. Institutions can be defined as the 'places' for the social organization of collective needs, and as such, they have the fundamental function of acting as an intermediate term between the reality of individuals and the structures of the organization of collective living and the economic-political power of a society (see Lynch, 2021). The theatre has been identified as a pivotal institution in the realm of community vitality and social participation, functioning as a crucible for the conceptualization of communal identity and the forging of social bonds. In this context, social participation can be considered an indicator of the potential for social cohesion, resistance, and transformation. This is particularly pertinent in the current era, where society is undergoing a gradual disruption from within, precipitated by the proliferation of social platforms and networks. These have the effect of fostering social interaction, but also concomitantly eroding social cohesion.

The chapter authored by Alex C. Michalos and P. Maurine Kahlke aims to measure the impact of arts-related activities on the perceived quality of life of a sample of British Columbians aged 18 years. This study was conducted during the spring of 2007 with the objective of comparing its results with those of a sample of 1,027 adults drawn from five B.C. communities (Comox Valley, Kamloops, Nanaimo, Port Moody and Prince George) collected in the fall of 2006. For the five communities considered, a comparison was made between all seven life assessment measures and self-assessed general health. It was found that self-assessed general health had the largest number of significant correlations with arts-related activities.

According to Arpad Szakolczai, theatre is a liminal genre that serves as an important conduit between societal factors and social transformation, with its historical evolution offering a substantial corpus of evidence concerning social processes and the status of society as a whole. The chapter's objective is to analyse in-depth three distinct case studies. Szakolczai's position is that these demonstrate theatre's function as a social indicator and catalyst. The author has selected Shakespeare, Molière, and Bulgakov as illustrative cases, with a view to demonstrating the capacity of theatre to reveal the 'state of soul' of a society, whilst simultaneously infecting society with mimetic desire, akin to the way a parasite infects. The phenomenon under discussion is exemplary of a mutual interplay or interference between an indicator and an agent. This is a characteristic inherent to all media.

Paolo Corvo's endeavour is to examine the particularities of Hamlet's character from a standpoint that transcends the boundaries of the immediate narrative, thereby ascertaining an abstract, universally relevant essence. Corvo's analysis employs a range of prominent sociological theories to contextualize Hamlet, drawing upon Erving Goffman's concept of life as play, Zygmunt Bauman's notion of a liquid society, and Anthony Giddens' theory of the crisis of modernity. This perspective draws upon seminal works such as those of Weber, providing a foundation for the exploration of contemporary issues. This essay seeks to demonstrate how Shakespeare imprinted society profoundly on one of his most significant works, thus illustrating the enduring influence of social forces on artistic expression.

The chapter by Alessandro Porrovecchio first explores key theoretical foundations of dramatherapy, emphasizing its potential to foster both individual and collective change. It then examines its practical applications within the framework of clinical sociology, drawing on our action-research projects.

The second part of the chapter presents three case studies. The first focuses on the ECAD (Expression Corporelle Adaptée et Désengagement Scolaire—Adapted Body Expression and School Disengagement) project and the doctoral research that followed, investigating how dramatherapy techniques can help students develop self-confidence and social integration in educational settings. The second case study explores dramatherapy among pre-bariatric patients, examining how theatrical methods contribute to reshaping body image perceptions, addressing emotional eating, and enhancing psychological well-being in individuals preparing for weight-loss surgery. The final case study delves into dramatherapy interventions with individuals affected by rare diseases, specifically Myasthenia Gravis, illustrating how the performative space enables participants to articulate their embodied experiences of illness and reimagine their identities beyond the constraints of medical narratives.

In the next chapter, Ulrike Loch seeks to elucidate the potential of theatre to engender shifts in collective memory with respect to the processing of violence. The article is grounded in the research project 'Gewalt an Kärntner Kindern und Jugendlichen in Institutionen' (Loch et al. 2022), which examines violence against children and adolescents within the framework of external placements and curative psychiatric childcare. The objective of this study is to examine the potential of collaborative endeavours between the social sciences and theatre to enhance the quality of life within a society that has been adversely affected by the repercussions of violence and associated taboo subjects, by modifying collective memory.

The chapter by Moreno Zago aims to examine the training needs within the performing, visual and live performance sectors, as well as the appeal and market requirements for such training. The case study selected is that of the Autonomous Region of Friuli-Venezia Giulia. In 2019, the region, with financial support from the European Social Fund, initiated the establishment of a Creative Cultural Technical Professional Pole with the objective to facilitate the coordination of educational and training programmes at the territorial level, integrating technical institutes, professional institutes, and vocational education and training courses. These programmes were designed to align with the training requirements of production processes and to be integrated with the economic and production systems.

The chapter by Laia Falcón deals with the theme of Covid pandemic trauma and how more than ever, theatre performances have become a source of well-being and quality of life. The chapter focuses on the case of ON AIR, staged in Madrid and Sevilla in 2020 as a revision of Orson Welles and Cole Porter's musical theatre piece Around the World. As a complementary revision of Welles and Porter's piece, with close ties to the prevailing social context of the pandemic and the emergent necessity for 'security proximity', the performance entitled ON AIR had its inaugural presentation in Madrid's National Concert Hall during the initial weeks following the imposition of confinement. The audience, the performers, and the critics all underscored the performance as a profoundly cathartic and well-being-promoting experience. The following observations provide substantiating evidence that collective experiences, such as attending a theatrical performance, can exert a significant influence on the imaginative faculties of the audience.

In Marxiano Melotti's chapter, the case of Terceira Carnival is examined. The analysis demonstrates the significant impact of theatre on the quality of life within a community, highlighting its role as a cultural institution with a profound influence on the local community's well-being. Terceira, an island in the Azores archipelago (Portugal), hosts a distinctive carnival celebration, bearing little resemblance to any other European carnival. In this context, masks and carnival floats are predominantly replaced by theatrical shows, which are both written and prepared by and for the local community and subsequently performed. This festival is a grassroots expression of the island's popular creativity, with significant identity implications for the island and its communities. It contributes to the definition and confirmation of relationships among the different villages on the island itself, as well as with the capital and the nation of the continent and the global context, through a complex interplay between centre and periphery, local and global, on different levels.

In her chapter, Maria Grazia Panigada tries to answer these questions: What are the implications of conceiving and designing a prose season? What are the steps to be followed, and what balances must be respected to create a theatre programme?

From a long time audience development studies have been warning us that putting different audiences at the centre of one's vision and of one's own way of creating culture, is definitely a winning strategy to increase the number of spectators. Above all, it is a way to make theatre a place that promotes the cultural life of the city and its territory. Through the «Stagione dei Teatri» (Theaters' Season) of the Fondazione Teatro Donizetti in Bergamo, an exemplary case will be presented, of how the quality of the proposal and the audience's training and education cause, as a primary consequence, the constant increase in the public and subscribers. In particular, the cultural policies and choices made will be presented, as they permitted to expand, diversify, and promote the active dimension of audiences, starting with the younger generations.

The chapter by Carlo Roncaglia deals with the function of the theatre director in the context of theatrical performance and the enhancement of the quality of life. The role of the theatre director in contemporary society is a delicate one—writes Roncaglia—requiring the ability to interpret and translate the constant changes in social and cultural life into artistic expression. Another salient aspect pertains to the responsibilities of the director in relation to the audience, who anticipates a positive stimulus for their quality of life from the theatrical performance. Carlo Roncaglia is a director and trainer who manages the theatre company 'Accademia dei Folli' in Turin. This chapter is concerned with the details of the work of a theatre director in contemporary society, with particular reference to the relationship with actors and the audience.

In his chapter, Mario Bois presents his personal experience of acting and theatre training as a means of facilitating self-knowledge and improved interpersonal relationships. He is an actor who is still at the beginning of his career, but he also works as a trainer. He is enthusiastic and committed to his work, and runs courses for children, young people, and adults. For a considerable duration, he has been engaged in the act of imparting knowledge and, in a broader sense, providing guidance to individuals on their journey towards significant revelations. Furthermore, he was able to discern the initial changes in their lives and the subsequent improvement in their well-being. The focus was not on the performance itself, nor on the audience. The issue at hand was not the clapping. The focus of these individuals was on their own development and the acquisition of knowledge.

The thematic elements identified in the various chapters of this book provide further evidence of the enduring significance of theatre as a crucial form of expression in and for contemporary societies, and as a means of promoting well-being in a virtual and globalized society.

Free University of Bolzano-Bozen
Bolzano BZ, Italy

Ilaria Riccioni
Ilaria.Riccioni@unibz.it

Contents

Part I
Structures

Chapter 1
Theatre as an Indicator for Social Participation and Well-being in Contemporary Western Societies

Ilaria Riccioni

Introduction

In what ways can artistic processes promote well-being in society? All artistic phenomena mediate the socio-political transformations taking place in the contemporary global world, as they provide a means for a society to reflect on itself. In contemporary times, individual actions are increasingly disjointed yet united by the same imagery. These actions are 'affectively oriented' and oscillate between politics and society, relying on imaginary communities defined by social platforms. In this uncertain balance, it is essential to understand the connection between the value dimensions and the emotional and affective load they carry in relation to socio-political and cultural institutions. While it is true that individuals are now asked for more emotional and irrational reactions than in previous times, due to the rapidity of virtual reality and the ephemeral nature of the metaverse, the antidote to such a loss can be found in theatre, which stages models of imagined reality.

According to Friedrich Nietzsche the birth of Western theatre, in the form of Greek tragedy, was deeply connected to the spirit of music. At the heart of theatre is an emotional language that speaks of things society often dares not reveal. It was in the Dionysian theatre that myths first emerged, uniting the collective imagination. As Nietzsche writes: 'To recognise that everything born must die, we must face the horrors of individual existence without being petrified. A metaphysical consolation instantly delivers us from the bustle of the ever-changing world. For a brief moment, we become the Primeval Being itself, experiencing its intense desire for and pleasure in existence' (Nietzsche, 1994: 111). In a tragedy, people can recognise themselves and reflect on their own condition: the importance of classical tragedy lies in

I. Riccioni (✉)
Free University of Bolzano-Bozen, Bolzano, Italy
e-mail: Ilaria.Riccioni@unibz.it

P. Corvo, I. Riccioni (eds.), *Theatre and Quality of Life*, Social Indicators Research Series 91, https://doi.org/10.1007/978-3-032-09731-6_1

its ability to let a society understand the bounds of reason (Nietzsche, 1994) but also to discover its condition of unity and collective destiny.

So, some of the indicators of social participation and community vitality can be found in the epic theatre as a core of imaginary and cultural creation of community belonging and theatre can be viewed as both a process and an institution that leads and organises social needs.

Institutions are the ‘places’ for the social organisation of collective needs, and as such they have the fundamental function of acting as an intermediate term between the reality of individuals and the structures of the organisation of collective living and the economic-political power of a society (see Lynch, 2021). So, some of the indicators of social participation and community vitality can be found in the epic theatre as core of imaginary and cultural creation of community belonging.

Here, social participation is intended as an indicator of the potential for social cohesion, resistance, and transformation in a relational society at a time when society is slowly being disrupted from within due to social platforms and networks that encourage social interaction but also erode it.

The Urgency and Obstacles of Research on the Arts and Theatre

In the two-volume book *Theatre and Social Sphere* (Brill), which I edited in 2023, the preface began with a consideration of how understanding and applying solutions to many social issues can be approached from new perspectives, such as a sociological understanding of the arts—in this case, theatre—and its relationship to its context: ‘The urgency to understand social dynamics in relation to their deeper motives, which include not only economic and normative needs, but also the fundamental human and social need for artistic and cultural forms that can foster coexistence and give it meaning, thereby improving quality of life. Artistic and cultural forms, as imaginative forms of collective social practices, fundamentally contribute to the meaning of a territory, context and people, as well as the generations who traverse these cultures’ (Riccioni, 2023: vii).

However, the study of theatre still faces many obstacles, as Maria Shevtsova clearly states: ‘The problem lies in the narrow and inadequate perception, conception, understanding and experience of what constitutes theatre. Theatre is not theatre unless it thoroughly embraces what is performed. The latter involves performance, which is intrinsic to theatre; otherwise, “theatre” remains a dramatic text while “performance” is adopted by discourses outside of theatre, where it serves as an analogy for social behaviours or a metaphor for social structures and apparent social influences’ (Shevtsova, 2023, p. 2). Therefore, when studying theatre as an indicator of social well-being or quality of life, the issue must be considered in terms of the wider arts. Both the text and the performance are, in a sense, the embodiment of the habitus of certain contexts. That said, the question of whether theatre can promote well-being must be explored through theatre itself, as well as the environment and context in which the performance takes place. In recent years, there has been a growing interest in prevention in Western countries.

Health issues for an ageing population are becoming a central commitment for many health institutions, as well as for Western governments, with an increase in research projects and funding in this area. Health and well-being have become a popular research topic, offering new perspectives on ageing and healthcare policies. The World Health Organization also writes in this vein, stating that 'Artistic expression grew in lockstep with human cultural development and has long played an integral part in how we teach, learn, communicate and heal'. Since our earliest ancestors began telling stories to make sense of the world, we have evolved to learn from narratives, whether through visual media, song, or performance.

The arts are uniquely suited to help us understand and communicate concepts and emotions by drawing on all our senses and our capacity for empathy. In recent decades, we have come to understand the intrinsic health benefits of artistic and leisure activities. Art can help us to emotionally navigate the journey of battling an illness or injury and to process difficult emotions in times of emergency and challenging events. The creation and enjoyment of the arts help promote holistic wellness and can be a motivating factor in recovery. Including the arts in health care delivery has been shown to support positive clinical outcomes for patients while also supporting other stakeholders, including health care providers, the patient's loved ones, and the wider community. Benefits are seen across several markers, including health promotion, the management of health conditions and illness, and disease prevention. As a matter of fact, the 1947 Constitution of the World Health Organization states, 'Health is a state of complete physical, mental, and social well-being and not merely the absence of disease or infirmity'. And with this in mind, WHO affirms that it has long used the arts in its work on health promotion and communication. Studies, especially anthropology, have shown that in early human history, art, religion and healing evolved in the same social space.

Also, research by the WHO Regional Office for Europe has shown that the use of artistic media in health care and in communities can have a variety of benefits for health outcomes. They can be used to communicate valuable messages across cultures and political divides, help affected communities understand the risks of certain diseases or behaviours, and provide ways for affected populations to process and learn from their individual and collective experience to improve their well-being among other benefits.

In accordance with these statements in 2019, WHO began testing arts interventions to advance specific health goals, including universal health coverage (UHC), mental health and suicide prevention, maternal health, blindness prevention and quality of care, in addition to historic efforts in HIV/AIDS prevention.

Collaborations with global media companies provide local-language programming on health issues in many areas of the world.

Over the past two decades, innovations incorporating the arts and health have been used to enhance physical and emotional support for resilience and well-being in communities, complementing and supporting therapeutic, rehabilitative, and preventive efforts, increasing awareness of health and contributing to emergency preparedness. WHO's Regional Office for Europe is leading work on research on the effect of art in health through its Behavioural and Cultural Insights Program.

As already mentioned before, this trend has taken over also the idea itself of orienting research on a European level. All Horizon research project funding for 2023–2027 is expressively dedicated to this area of research development, especially in European countries, and this is a sign of a renewed attention on how cultural heritage, cultural practices, and artistic expressions in all their different ways, such as music, performance, theatre, but also visual arts, are deeply involved in the development and the well-being of a country. As a matter of fact, also cognitive sciences have provided evidence of a direct link between well-being, cognitive development, and cultural experience.

Many countries have acknowledged the power of cultural resources. The Ottawa Charter for Health Promotion, drafted already in 1986, was the outcome of the First International Conference on Health Promotion, which took place in Ottawa in November of that same year. This charter emphasised the importance of taking action to achieve Health for All by the year 2000 and beyond. This conference was primarily in response to the growing expectation of a new public health movement worldwide. While discussions focused on the needs of industrialised countries, similar concerns in other regions were also taken into account. It is also the result of the combined progress made through the 1978 Alma-Ata Declaration on Primary Health Care, the World Health Organization's Health for All targets, and the recent debate at the World Health Assembly on intersectoral action for health.

Health promotion is a process of potentially enabling people to increase their control over and improve their health.

In order to achieve a state of complete physical, mental, and social well-being, individuals or groups must be able to identify and realise their aspirations, satisfy their needs, and change or cope with their environment.

Therefore, health is seen as a resource for everyday life, rather than an end in itself. It is a positive concept that emphasises social and personal resources, as well as physical capacities.

Therefore, health promotion is not only the responsibility of the health sector; it goes beyond healthy lifestyles to encompass well-being, which also implies a mind–body–society equilibrium that can be cultivated through arts and cultural experiences, which are recognised to be part of a good, wise, and satisfying life.

According to the WHO the prerequisites for health are mostly in relation to the quality of life and therefore directly imply the societal structure in which citizens are embedded. As a consequence the fundamental conditions and resources for health are recognised as fundamental as follows:

- peace,
- shelter,
- education,
- food,
- income,

- a stable ecosystem,
- sustainable resources,
- social justice, and equity.

Any improvement in health requires a secure foundation in these basic prerequisites—writes WHO in its site—so the issue of health has exited the pure physical condition to become a wider concept embracing the environment and quality of social relations in which good health turns out to be a major resource for social, economic, and personal development, therefore a fundamental dimension of a quality of life. Political, economic, social, cultural, environmental, behavioural, and biological factors can all favour health or be harmful to it. The aim of health promotion action is to create favourable conditions through health advocacy. In this sense, demographic data illustrate the significant differences in life expectancy between developed and developing countries.

Arts, Health, and Well-being

Studies have shown that art and activities based on art have diverse positive impacts on physical health, mental well-being as well as perceived well-being, quality of life, and happiness. There is evidence that the context of living is responsible for:

- Improving the results of medical treatment and alleviating physical and psychological symptoms;
- Reducing the need and use of anxiolytic medication, painkillers, and sleeping pills;
- Helping alleviate loneliness and social isolation;
- Preventing and reducing negative emotions, such as anxiety, depression, and sadness; and,
- Helping people cope with mental health issues.

In addition, each person has the right to take part in arts and culture, to develop themselves and their community through arts and culture, and to express themselves freely.

These cultural rights are stipulated in the Universal Declaration of Human Rights adopted by the UN (1948) (Taikusydan Arts & Health Coordination Centre in Finland, 2019).

Since 2009, the journal Arts & Health has provided a pioneering international forum for the publication of research, policy, and best practice within the *interdisciplinary field of arts and health.*

This fast-emerging field has developed in response to international interest regarding the multifarious ways in which the arts contribute to health, well-being, social inclusion, and healthcare practice across a range of settings.

The field has become an inter- and multi-disciplinary arena for those concerned with research, policy, and practice initiatives, including artists, healthcare professionals, community workers, and researchers in the public, private, and voluntary sectors.

The field of arts in health research is currently undergoing a burgeoning of activity (Fancourt & Finn, 2019).

There are increasing numbers of research reports being published in journals ranging from the arts to medicine, nursing, rehabilitation, psychology, the arts therapies, neuroscience, biology, and technology.

There are a growing number of international conferences on the topic, including the yearly Global Alliance for Arts and Health conference, which began in 1989; the International Conference for Culture, Health and Wellbeing in England, in June 2013; the International Arts and Health Conference in Australia, November 2013; and the International Association for Music and Medicine Conference in Canada, in June 2014.

Moreover, there are more and more associations growing all over Europe and the world as there is a new recognition of the importance of the holistic roots of well-being, which is more and more also a cultural affair, focused on understanding and creating a positive connection with the surroundings and its cultural meanings.

Arts and culture make a significant contribution to our health and well-being. In times of the coronavirus pandemic, this topic takes on even more urgency. Art and culture can play a positive role in both the management and prevention of (psychological, mental, and physical) stress and its consequences.

The 'Arts for Health' workshop organised by the BKA on 5 December 2019 was the first time this topic was discussed on a broad scale in Austria. Despite isolated, exemplary initiatives, there is still too little awareness in Austria overall, both in the cultural and health sectors, and hardly any structural approaches.

The association ARTS for HEALTH AUSTRIA (AfHA) for the promotion of art interventions in the context of health and well-being aims to remedy these structural deficits.

The association sees itself as a platform for art activities in the field of public health in Austria, as an interface between artists, researchers, and health institutions and as a national and international networking instrument and contact point for all those interested in this field.

Overall, the debate on art interventions in the healthcare sector in Austria is still in its initial stages. The initiatives of ARTS for HEALTH AUSTRIA are therefore based on the experiences of international institutions with the same objectives and orientation. The proponents of AfHA are well networked internationally and are willing to develop the association's activities in close cooperation with similar institutions.

The areas of responsibility of AfHA are:

- Providing a platform for art activities in the public health sector in Austria;
- Acting as interface between art and science;
- Building a national and international networking tool;
- Serving as an information point for all those interested in this area.
- Funding organization for innovative art projects in the healthcare sector.

Another evidence of disruption of the arts in everyday life practices is that of the so-called 'social prescribing': in Britain, Finland, Switzerland, and elsewhere, doctors can prescribe a patient a theatre subscription or a museum visit, given the recognition of such activities as forms of improving living conditions. The IBSA Foundation is an international non-profit organisation established in Lugano in 2012. Born from the Institut Biochimique, it aspires to promote research, disseminate scientific culture, and train young scholars through forums, workshops, scholarships, and publications. Moreover, it performs an active function that is intended to elevate the general consciousness of the public with regard to the notions of health, quality of life, and personal care, employing artistic communication as a medium.

The positive impact of the arts on health is now being increasingly recognised by governments around the world. In Australia, for example, the Federal, State, and Territory Ministers endorsed the National Arts and Health Policy Framework. And one example is the project carried out by Wollongong and Melbourne, Australia-based NGO Neami Community Art with a 20-years mental health art program. The project aims to use art as a rehabilitative method, creating employment opportunities and fostering independence for people with disabilities. It involves courses in various art disciplines for people currently living with mental health issues, with the aim of rehabilitating them and developing their artistic skills as a means of gaining a place in society.

The program supports individuals facing complex and enduring mental health challenges in developing an arts practice under the guidance of community artists. Through everyday arts studio sessions, participants can learn new skills, develop confidence, and forge connections through creative expression. The program also challenges the idea that art has value only as therapy, instead recognising that it can transform lives. Also, the US National Endowment for the Arts is working with federal agencies and providing funding for arts projects and research. The Finnish government departments for Health & Social Care and Education & Culture are also involved in creating projects to support the health of older adults through the arts; the All-Party Parliamentary Group on Arts and Health has also been established in the UK.

Based on a scoping review of over 3000 studies in several European countries, the WHO report of 2019 signed by Fancourt and Finn is the first dissemination document that demonstrates the effectiveness of specific cultural, artistic, and creative activities as a determining factor for:

(1) Health promotion, also related to the acquisition of coping skills and the development of life skills;
(2) Subjective well-being and satisfaction with life;
(3) Combating health inequalities and social cohesion by facilitating access to and development of individual and community social capital;
(4) Active ageing, combating depression and psychophysical decline resulting from neglect and isolation;

(5) Inclusion and empowerment for people with disabilities and for people in conditions of marginalisation or disadvantage;
(6) Complement to traditional therapeutic treatment;
(7) Support to the doctor–patient relationship, through medical humanities and the physical transformation of care places;
(8) Support to the care relationship, also and especially for non-professional carers;
(9) Management of some degenerative conditions, such as dementia and Parkinson's disease. However, there remains a problem surrounding research in this field:

'For researchers, there seems to be constant friction between selecting methods that meet the strict requirements of health research and methods that accurately capture the essence and impact of the art involved. For artists, scientific jargon can hinder the development of robust, publishable research studies, while for funders, arts in health can fall between the humanities and sciences, whose aims and methodologies may be unfamiliar to each other'. Fancourt and Finn continue: 'The crux of this problem lies in the fact that there is currently no reference point for arts in health research, and no standard for the development, design, delivery, or dissemination of such research projects'. (Fancourt & Finn, 2019).

Another development in the social dimension of arts and theatre is the concept of 'cultural welfare', which stems from the aforementioned recognition endorsed by the World Health Organization (Fancourt & Finn, 2019; Cicerchia et al., 2020). The WHO Report documents several specific and desirable impacts of theatre, both as an active practice (e.g. people who participate in laboratories, workshops, acting courses, etc.) and as a regular passive participation (going to the theatre and being a spectator of live acting performances). (Cicerchia & Staffieri, 2023). According to a more specific focus on the theatre, the line of Boal's Theatre of the Oppressed, which is working in detention camps for migrants, or in situations of disabilities (il teatro Patologico), it is very well known in Italy the improvement of everyday life that theatre has had when tested on prisoners. Since 2011 in Italy there is a formally recognised body, 'The National Coordination of Prison Theater', that aims at enhancing the experience of acting companies made up of prisoners who have been operating in various institutions for decades.

At the beginning of the initiative, which occurred 14 years ago, the Coordination involved 12 prisons. Presently, the initiative has expanded to involve more than 40 experiences across 14 Italian regions, with approximately 70 institutions participating in the activities. The protocol between the Coordination and the Italian Ministry of Justice dates back to 2013; With the signing of the document, the body began celebrating Prison Theater Day (March 27), which was also joined by Dance Day (April 29). A busy schedule of performances by inmate companies inside and outside institutions takes place between the two anniversaries. Vito Minoia, the President and founder of the National Coordination, has been involved in social theatre since his university studies in sociology at Urbino. His mentor was Emilio Pozzi, a renowned theatre historian who, after his death, was described by the Piccolo Teatro di Milano as a 'careful interpreter of the irreplaceable role of public theatre'. Minoia founded the magazine Catarsi—Theatres of Diversity with Pozzi in 1996.

Culture emerges, then, as a key variable in the development of the quality of life but also in the ability to respond to existential and pathological stresses by virtue of its ability to expand human capacities in terms of knowledge, regenerative resources and forms of creative solutions to the challenges of everyday life. The reasons why culture is so effective are yet to be understood, but it is perhaps fundamental to generate that capacity of being in the world that Simmel writes about (Simmel, 1968, 2020). For example, neuroscience tells us that culture defines 'allostasis': cultural experience enters into these allostatic regulatory processes, defining their ability to enhance emotional regulation and immune response and the capacity of our endocrine system to respond to certain or excessive levels of stress. This is evidence of culture's regulatory role in human survival and adaptation to changing life situations. Culture is a vital resource that enables people to cope with everyday and extraordinary challenges. In 2018, the new European agenda finally expressed the link between culture, health, and economy.

The European Community began to promote research themes through the Horizon Europe programme, which increasingly focuses on the relationship between culture and health. Even in 2023–2026, it remains one of the 21 key actions. Within the new ecosystem, culture and creativity, as well as the culture and health theme, play a central role. Europe is undergoing an epochal transition, and as a result, the theme of cultural welfare is taking on an unprecedentedly central role. In particular, new scenarios are unfolding in the field of social issues and in building more resilient societies, as well as in ensuring the sustainability of life in late modern societies. It also has revolutionary potential for the management of social policy. It can also encourage societies to become more aware of the well-being of their citizens, which is brought about by cultural experiences and not just economic resources. A relatively new approach that is gaining ground is Cultural Welfare, which 'indicates a new, integrated model for promoting the well-being and health of individuals and communities through practices involving the visual and performing arts, and cultural heritage' (Cicerchia & Staffieri, 2023: 186).

The Contextualised Culture of the Theatre as a Tool for Well-being

On another level, academic studies have been developing the core of these new achievements and there is always more research and attention to the social role of culture and emotions, as well as a justice-injustice interplay among societal dynamics. Many studies inquire into the social role of the arts, be it theatre, performance, painting, music, dancing, etc. or the agency of culture in widening personal horizons in terms of understanding a changing reality, such as cultural diversity, due to migrations, new needs, and widespread diversity brought about by the digital society.

In his inquiry into theatre, Tinius (2023) brings the example of the Theater an der Ruhr, a public repertory theatre ensemble based in the Ruhr Valley in North Rhine-Westphalia founded by Roberto Ciulli, an émigré philosopher and self-taught director who moved from Italy to Germany in the 1960s. This theatre is 'a theatre of and for the *Bastardo'*, meaning those without a fatherland or a mother tongue, aiming to challenge the predominant framing of cultural production through the category of the nation. (Tinius, 2023: 3).

The relevance of this theatre for a social perspective lies in the fact of being an exemplary contemporary German public theatre institution situated at the intersection of important German cultural and intellectual traditions, yet ethically and artistically committed to pursuing an alternative politics. On the one hand, this theatre challenges artistic conventions that expect actors to identify with their roles. On the other hand, it challenges the cultural identity of modern Germany. Tinius outlines a genealogy of *Bildung* in German history. *Bildung* is a concept of self-cultivation and self-realisation developed already by thinkers like Schiller, Schlegel, and Humboldt who were also involved in theatre. The core idea of Tinius is that *Bildung,* neither apolitical nor anti-political, promotes introspective self-criticism. It prioritises self-improvement over the care of others for the greater good. He contends that Theater an der Ruhr is a response to, not an extension of, Bildung traditions. The theatre's impact on a community is connected to its traditions and types of habitus, therefore embodying the essence of a contextualised culture and its critique (Tinius, 2023).

If I may add, the outcome of my research on the social impact of the state theatre in the Bolzano province showed that cultural institutions can play a central role in a community, not only in terms of culture, but also by fostering a sense of social belonging, socialisation, and identity, particularly in minority contexts (Riccioni, 2020).

Theatre is an evolving cultural institution whose role emerges mainly from its interaction with the community, rather than being predetermined. It is this interaction that determines its role and function. In the case of the Teatro Stabile in Bolzano, for example, the research results showed that its role is to promote inclusion and overcome divisive dynamics. It is a centre for the production and research of new cultural forms and collaborations, returning to citizens the idea of an institution as a community service and a place for personal growth. According to Duvignaud's theory of theatre as collective ceremony, theatre is enjoyed by some more than others. When this collective ceremony does not succeed, sociological inquiry should focus on three basic indicators: the relationship of theatre to its context, its capacity to reflect contemporary society, and its function as a catalyst for social participation (Duvignaud, 1965). These three elements are indeed indicators of social welfare, social cohesion, and ultimately civic awareness within a given context. They certainly indicate well-being on social rather than economic terms, cultural vitality, an inclination towards civic values and a tendency towards creativity. We would also venture towards the 'democratising' power of theatre and the resilience of culture.

A high number of references to the resilience capacities to which every cultural form tends to socialise were found in the data collected.

For theatre this potential is enhanced as it operates on value, cultural and personal dimensions in the direction of an emotional 'swing' that exercises the elaboration of emotions generating resilience capacity, acceptance of diversity as universality, the opening of horizons, which is part of everyone's life process. In other words, theatre brings the individual's experience back to a collective level and unveils our common challenges, difficulties, frustrations, and joys, and reintroduces these into the life stream through collective reflection (Riccioni, 2017, 2020). On the side of the institutional organisation this theatre is quite privileged exactly because of its peculiar context. In fact, it can rely on a solid financial statement that breaks even every year, which is quite exceptional among Italian theatres. In fact, it has the support of the Italian state, the Province and the city of Bolzano. The total sum is well administered, and the theatre itself can also count on a good number of subscriptions. All of this makes the Bolzano Theatre a thriving institution with solid financial foundations, as well as the capacity to produce innovative forms of relational and diffuse theatre, and to stage the works of the most prominent Italian authors.

An interesting empirical analysis of U.S. resident non-profit theatres and innovation, carried out by Paul DiMaggio and Kristen Stenberg already in 1985, reports that theatres with access to patrons rich in cultural capital appear to have more innovative repertoires, while dependence on the market (as opposed to grants and contributions) is associated with greater conformity of repertoire. Theatres with smaller budgets, fewer seats, and less need for earned income are less conformist in their programming than large theatres with high capacity and high earned income rates. When size and dependence on earned income are held constant, there is no evidence that age, structural differentiation, or the presence of subscription audiences—all of which are associated with 'institutionalisation'—have either a negative or positive impact on innovation. Theatres in New York innovate more and are less negatively affected by growth and the market than theatres elsewhere in the US. It is suggested that artistic innovation has come to depend overwhelmingly on the behaviour of formal organisations, as we might confirm in the case of the Theatre in Bolzano, for example, and consequently, artistic change and the capacity for innovation is strictly connected to the principles that govern the relationship of such organisations to their economic and social environments (DiMaggio & Stenberg, 1985). This also plays a significant role in the capacity of the arts and theatre to generate well-being for communities and societies.

Innovation, Creativity and the Construction of New Paradigms

What is creativity and what is its role within social structure and everyday life coping strategies, as well as its role in social well-being. As I reflected upon in an article dedicated to creativity in 2008, creativity can be defined as the capacity to see beyond the empirical data of reality. The artist, through the use of metaphor, can be considered a self-exile who maintains contact with an over-reality, thus creating a universal world from small, everyday events. This capacity for creating is, in a certain way, the merging of the elaborated experience and the use of imaginary processes, and can be considered the only possibility for a society to produce innovation. Innovation in itself cannot emerge from nothing, according to the axiom of Lavoisier: 'In nature nothing is destroyed and nothing is created from nothing, but everything is being transformed'.

In a totally organised and bureaucratised society, as Horkheimer called it, creativity is the element that provokes disorder and may act as a blocking agent to all the organised social system, enhancing change and proposing innovative and more adequate styles of life (Riccioni, 2008). Although that article did not explore the various ways in which creativity can manifest itself in everyday life, I already had a clear understanding of how the everyday experience of creativity is often undervalued. Indeed, studies have focused on the different manifestations of creativity and its diverse effects on everyday life. This has led to the acknowledgement of a gender divide in creativity, with innovative, male-dominated creativity being recognised more readily than less recognised forms of creativity involving a more collaborative and environmental approach: 'the term creativity, rather than just innovativeness, would be reserved for that which supports, nurtures, and actualises life by increasing the number of choices open to individuals and communities. It would therefore not be applied to the development of technologies that kill. Nor would it be applied to the development of better means of dominating, exploiting, and/or limiting the choices available to people' (Eisler, Donnelly & Montuori, 2016: 25). In fact, the issue of creativity is closely connected to the issue of innovation that was mentioned earlier. However, distinguishing between these two concepts makes it possible to introduce a third concept that is crucial in social dynamics: the ethical dimension of creativity.

Many creativity scholars have claimed for an ethical consideration of creativity: some of them such as Barron (1988), Gruber (1988), and McLaren (1993) have emphasised the importance of addressing urgent social issues through creativity, while also emphasised that creativity can have different outcomes. 'McLaren, for example, has discussed "the dark side of creativity", highlighting the nature of what he terms "destructive creativity" in close parallel to Eisler's "technologies of destruction"' (McLaren, 1993).

Loye has called for 'moral creativity', distinguishing between a 'dominator morality' of coercion and a 'partnership morality' of caring. And Richard Kearney (1999) has argued that humans have an ethical demand to imagine otherwise; in other words, to go beyond what is to what could be and, indeed, what should be. (Eisler, Donnelly & Montuori, 2016: 26). It is also by framing theatre as an 'extraordinary' field of ethical reflection (Tinius, 2023) that this complex, articulate art form, which is grounded in and engages with everyday life experiences, can contribute to theoretical discussions about how the arts can provide a privileged platform for politics, society, and intellectual thought. There is, however, a gender approach to creativity that suggests that 'Creative approaches to problems in communities, reflect the movement in the research literature to the social, every-day, "ordinary" and collaborative dimensions of creativity'. (p. 26). According to Arieti (1976), societies have a 'creativogenic' nature, implying the capacity for communities to self-organise and address problems creatively. However, this capacity for self-organisation is rooted in the relational and enabling skills that women have traditionally been socialised to possess to a greater extent than men, alongside their contextual focus. A society capable of making creativity a resource for social issues is also capable of finding positive solutions to its problems and developing a collaborative approach to emerging issues that can be synthesised in a way of acting that gives birth to something that was not there before (Popitz, 2000: 98). In other words, creativity has to do with imagination but is much more than that: it is the ability that only human beings have to 'das Seiende außerhalb seiner selbst als ein Anderssein, als eigenartiges So-Sein zu erfassen' (Popitz, 2000: 98–99). This opens up new challenges and new paradigms that need to be fine-tuned.

Art, Theatre and the Idea of the Other

Already in the book Theatre and Public Sphere I have been inquiring how theatre today can play a role in the contemporary loss of belonging and meaning in modern societies, and through the recovery of the presence, the link between body and mind can reorganise everyday life around experience ((Riccioni, 2023: vii) According to Maria Shevtsova 'In the practice of the theatre, sign-making signs are meaningful because people makes them in socialised contexts in the social world. They do not function within a self-enclosed and self-explanatory system abstracted from the social world (the focus of systemic theories). Signs are carriers of the socially saturated meanings inscribed in social action, and they carry into the imagined, fictional worlds of theatres. Reconfigured, they nevertheless make sense, have impact, affect emotions, and stimulate imagination and thought. This is precisely how the "outside" world comes into the "inside" of theatre worlds.

It is precisely how and why social contexts, although specified differently in different theatre performances, are always inside those performances and discernible in them (…) Since social contexts are embodied within artistic processes, claims that they are merely backgrounds, exterior to the art forms at issue, seriously need to be questioned, first and foremost in theatre scholarship, where old dualistic habits die hard—aleatory "background" contra real-deal theatre at the foreground. Even so, the issue is not one of seeking and finding exact replicas of corresponding social contexts in the semioses of theatre works'. (Shevtsova, 2023). In postmodern societies, cultural institutions such as museums and theatres play an unprecedented role: they are rediscovered as places where collective needs are intercepted, responded to and organised (see also Riccioni, 2021). With the end of the time of cultural institutions as elite places, these particular institutions have taken on a radical relational and pedagogical change of direction. Theatres also seem to respond to this need for institutions to open up to all kinds of audience, bringing the pedagogical energies and strategies of other structures into play.

In addition, the theatre is a place of aggregation for young and adult generations for different reasons, the former theatre is a place to learn emotions, collective work and collaboration in person, thus overcoming the dangers posed by high exposure to digital devices; for the latter instead, having been formed through reflection and the social commitment of theatre, is a place of aggregation, of social resistance and celebration. (Riccioni, 2023: 20). For example The mission of Swiss director Milo Rau and his team, who, in several Central African countries (The Democratic Republic of the Congo, Rwanda, and Burundi), have created theatre largely with non-actors and/or some aspiring actors. (…) Rau concentrates and then diffuses his socio-political drive, embracing like-driven aspirant performers as well as spectators to make theatre that is social through and through. This theatre, which is steeped in current affairs and daily language, and relies on verbatim-theatre, documentary, reportage, courtroom examination and other legal-procedural techniques as it probes social realities, could, indeed, be described as sociological theatre.

And this suggests that theatre, when it is like Rau's, is another way of doing sociology. The Rau-group theatre is an agitprop theatre with unambiguous, fully explicit signifying through which the distinctions between theatre and life are erased, as is the very idea of theatre as make-believe. The theatre-act enacts and incarnates social justice—hence the idea of the tribunal, the means by which the first steps to justice can be secured; and enactment, incarnation, and tribunal endorsement, as well as moral confirmation, promote the necessity of social justice in reality, not in fiction. (…) Here, life itself, understood as exploitation and corruption, is the theatre of requisite radical transformation, and this life is nothing if not public and political through and through. (Shevtsova, 2023: 6).

Temporary Conclusions

In a recent interview, Alicia Giménez-Bartlett, Spain's leading mystery novelist, revealed the secrets behind her books. She describes writing as a form of self-therapy that enables her to create a reality in which life becomes bearable. This is the transformative power of being fascinated by the imaginary worlds of novels. She emphasises that this is particularly important during challenging periods, stating that 'writing can become therapy'. The well-being that art offers stems from its capacity to stimulate the imagination and provide a vision that opens up potentialities for a better world, life or society. 'Visual, performing, and media arts have—writes Paltrinieri—the "power" to give "power", that is, to develop forms of "agency", to empower their audiences by leveraging their attractive nature' (Paltrinieri & Spampinato, 2024) and in fact, art can disrupt the established order, leading to a new one. Creativity offers different perspectives to those commonly established in society.

In this way, art can rediscover reality. The moment of reinvention is mysterious, when the mundane connects with the universal, but its outcome becomes the manifestation of a need, which is mostly a collective need. Both Duvignaud (1965) and Durkheim (1912–2008) affirm that a society's custom of attending collective events lies in the emotions of belonging that such events evoke. In this sense, although with different connotations, Badiou also defines the concept of 'event' as the richness of the collective experience offered by theatre (Badiou, 2013). Theatre generates an event, an occurrence: it activates reflection and the interplay between thought and feeling, which reconfigures daily life through the centrality of the body, understood as the unity of experience. Experience is the element that attracts, captures, and affiliates the spectator to the theatre. In an increasingly digitised society where opportunities for experience are being replaced by screens and artificial intelligence, theatre provides evidence that it can be a place to reconnect with humanity's collective experience as a primary source of well-being.

References

Arieti, S. (1976). *Creativity: The Magic Synthesis*. New York: Basic Books.

Badiou, A. (2013). *Rhapsody for the theatre*. Verso.

Barron, F. (1988). *Putting creativity to work*. In R. Sternberg (Ed.), The nature of creativity (pp. 76–98). Cambridge: Cambridge University Press.

Cicerchia, A., Rossi-Ghiglione, A., & Seia, C. (2020). *Welfare culturale*. Atlante Treccani della Cultura.

Cicerchia, A., & Staffieri, S. (2023). Cultural welfare. Theatre in the limelight. In I. Riccioni (Ed.), *Theatre(s) and public sphere in a digital and global society (Vol. 1) "theoretical explorations"* (pp. 186–196). Brill.

DiMaggio, P., & Stenberg, K. (1985). Why do some theatres innovate more than others? An empirical analysis. *Poetics, 14*(1–2), 107–122.

Durkheim, É. (1912–2008). *The elementary forms of religious life*. OUP.

Duvignaud, J. (1965). *Sociologie du Théâtre. Essai sur les ombres collectives*. PUF.

Eisler, R., Donnelly, G., & Montuori, A. (2016). Creativity, society, and gender: Contextualizing and redefining creativity. *Interdisciplinary Journal of Partnership Studies, 3*(2), 3. http://pubs.lib.umn.edu/ijps/vol3/iss2/3

Fancourt, D., & Finn, S. (2019). What is the evidence on the role of the arts in improving health and Well-being? A scoping review. WHO. Health Evidence Network synthesis report 67. https://www.who.int/europe/publications/i/item/9789289054553

Gruber, H. E. (1988). *The evolving systems approach to creative work. Creativity Research Journal, 1*, 27–51. https://doi.org/10.1080/10400418809534285

Kearney, R. (1999). The narrative imagination. In A. Montuori & R. Purser (Eds.), *Social creativity* (Vol. 1, pp. 61–79). Hampton Press.

Lynch, K. (2021). Affective equality and social justice. In D. Celentano & L. Caranti (Eds.), *Paradigms of justice*. Routledge.

McLaren, R. B. (1993). The dark side of creativity. *Creativity Research Journal, 6*(1–2), 137–144.
Montuori, A., & Donnelly, G. (2016). The creativity of culture and the culture of creativity research: The promise of integrative transdisciplinarity. In V. P. Glăveanu (Ed.), *The Palgrave handbook of creativity and culture research* (pp. 743–765). Palgrave Macmillan/Springer Nature. https://doi.org/10.1057/978-1-137-46344-9_36
Nietzsche, F. (1994). *The birth of tragedy: Out of the spirit of music*. Penguin Classics.
Paltrinieri, R., & Spampinato, F. (2024). *Arte come Agency. Il valore sociale e politico delle arti nelle comunità*. Franco Angeli.
Popitz, H. (2000). *Wege der Kreativität*. Tübingen: Mohr Siebeck.
Riccioni, I. (2008). Art and creativity. *CULTURA21* – online journal.
Riccioni, I. (2017). I fondamenti relazionali e sociologici del teatro. In *Rivista Metis* (Vol. XXIV, No. 1, pp. 177–200). Cleup.
Riccioni, I. (2020). *Teatro e Società: il caso dello stabile di Bolzano*. Carocci.
Riccioni, I. (2021). The social turn of institutions: Museums as social spaces, memory builders and social discourse stimulants. In E. Polyudova (Ed.), *Arts museums in modern society* (pp. 34–54). Cambridge Scholars Publishing.
Riccioni, I. (Ed.). (2023). *Theatre(s) and public sphere in a global and digital society. Theoretical Explorations. Vol. 1* (Studies in critical social sciences series). Brill.
Shevtsova, M. (2023). Artistic processes and characteristics: Key problems of the sociology of the theatre. In dialogue with Pierre Bourdieu. In I. Riccioni (Ed.), *Theatre(s) and public sphere in a global and digital society. Theoretical explorations (Vol. 1)* (Studies in critical social sciences series). Brill.
Simmel, G. (1968). *The conflict in modern culture and other essays*. Teachers College Press.
Simmel, G. (2020). *Essays on art and aesthetics*. University of Chicago Press.
Tinius, J. (2023). *State of the arts: An ethnography of German theatre and migration*. Cambridge University Press.

Chapter 2
Arts and the Perceived Quality of Life in British Columbia

Alex C. Michalos and P. Maurine Kahlke

Sampling Technique and Questionnaire

The 13-page questionnaire used in the survey undertaken for this investigation was a revised version of one used for the five-community survey described in Michalos and Kahlke (2008). In May 2007, 5000 questionnaires were mailed out to a random sample of households across the whole province of British Columbia. The first three pages of the questionnaire listed 66 activities that are related in one way or another to the arts, e.g., listening to music, teaching painting or drawing, singing in a group, attending live theatre performances. Because people participate in different artistic activities in very different time periods, from daily (e.g., listening to music) to a few times per year (e.g., attending live theatre performances), to properly estimate the amount of time committed to such activities, two different questions were included. For activities involving frequent participation, respondents were asked to estimate the average amount of time per week that they spent on them, in hours. If they never engaged in some particular activity, they were asked to write 0 for hours per week. For activities involving infrequent participation, respondents were asked to estimate the number of times per year that they participated in them. If they never engaged in some particular activity, they were asked to write 0 for times per year. For those activities in which they participated, they were asked to rate the average level of satisfaction obtained on a 7-point scale running from 1 = very dissatisfied, 2 or 3 = dissatisfied, 4 = even balance of satisfaction and dissatisfaction, 5 or

A. C. Michalos (✉)
University of Northern British Columbia, Prince George, BC, Canada
e-mail: michalos@unbc.ca

P. M. Kahlke
Institute for Social Research and Evaluation (ISRE), University of Northern British Columbia, Prince George, BC, Canada
e-mail: hatchp@unbc.ca

P. Corvo, I. Riccioni (eds.), *Theatre and Quality of Life*, Social Indicators Research Series 91, https://doi.org/10.1007/978-3-032-09731-6_2

6 = satisfied, to 7 = very satisfied. The Appendix attached to this paper has a complete list of all the activities sorted and ordered by (1) the numbers of people participating in each, (2) the average number of hours per week people engaged in each and (3) the average number of times per year that people engaged in each. Copies of the questionnaire and detailed responses to all items are available from the corresponding author on request.

Following the frequency-of-participation items, there was a page of questions designed to get more information about the arts-related activity (out of the 66) that respondents perceived as 'most important'. For example, there were questions about levels of satisfaction with their access to the activity, with the price of engagement and with the usual venue, and questions about where they first learned about the activity, e.g., in school, watching television, listening to a friend and how old they were at the time.

The next two pages listed 45 statements culled from the literature describing people's beliefs and feelings about the arts, usually phrased in personal terms, e.g., My artistic activities help me preserve my cultural heritage, I engage in artistic activities to express my spirituality, I enjoy art for its own sake. Sometimes the phrasing was impersonal, e.g., Artistic activity strengthens a community, Good art needs no justification beyond itself. Respondents were given a 5-point Likert scale and asked to indicate for each item their level of agreement or disagreement, with strongly disagree = 1 and strongly agree = 5.

There were then two pages of standard questions about respondents' health and quality of life. These included questions about life as a whole and about specific domains and aspects of life, e.g., family relations, friendships, sense of meaning in life. Seven overall assessments of life were used as dependent variables in this study: (1) self-reported general health using a 5-point scale from poor to excellent, (2) satisfaction with life as a whole using a 7-point scale from very dissatisfied to very satisfied, (3) satisfaction with the overall quality of life using a 7-point scale from very dissatisfied to very satisfied, (4) happiness with life as a whole using a 7-point scale from very unhappy to very happy, (5) satisfaction with life as a whole using a 5-item index drawn from Diener et al. (1985), (6) contentment with life using a 5-item index drawn from Lavallee et al. (2007) and (7) subjective wellbeing using a 4-item index (Michalos et al., 2005). All measures of satisfaction with particular domains or aspects of life were formatted as 7-point scales running from very dissatisfied to very satisfied and these measures have been used around the world for over 30 years (Michalos, 2005a).

Following these standard questions, there were two pages of questions designed to test some of the basic hypotheses of Multiple Discrepancies Theory (MDT, Michalos, 1985), e.g., Considering your life as a whole, how does it measure up to your general aspirations or what you want out of life? How does it measure up to the best in your previous experience? This is only the second survey allowing some testing of MDT in the context of a wide variety of information about arts-related activities and the perceived quality of life.

Finally, there were 2 pages of demographic questions about, e.g., age, sex, marital status, income and education.

Sample Characteristics

A total of 708 (14.2%) useable questionnaires were returned, which form the working data set for the survey. Table 2.1 summarizes the main features of the respondent sample.

The first substantive column of the table lists statistics for the unweighted sample, the second lists those statistics weighted by age and education according to the census of 2006 and the final column lists the 2006 census values for comparative purposes. All of our analyses are based on the weighted sample.

Table 2.1 Sample demographics, unweighted and weighted numbers and % and census (Statistics Canada, 2006 Census Data) values, numbers and %

	Unweighted		Weighted		Census values	
Characteristic	N	%	N	%	N	%
Gender • Female	455	65.7	457	65.9	1,745,320	51.4
• Male	238	34.3	236	34.1	1,649,585	48.6
Total	693	100.0	693	100.0	3,394,905	100.0
Age • 20–34	86	12.4	167	24.2	762,435	24.4
• 35–44	140	20.3	137	19.9	622,615	19.9
• 45–54	165	23.9	146	21.1	661,485	21.2
• 55–64	167	24.2	113	16.4	502,645	16.2
• 65 and over	133	19.2	127	18.4	572,420	18.3
Total	691	100.0	690	100.0	3,121,600	100.0
Education—highest level Secondary—incomplete	32	4.7	110	16.0	502,270	16.1
• Secondary—complete	165	24.0	189	27.5	858,115	27.5
• Diploma, certificate, etc.	165	24.0	205	29.7	924,820	29.6
• Some university	100	14.5	40	5.8	182,695	5.9
• University degree	226	32.8	144	21.0	653,700	20.9
Total	688	100.0	688	100.0	3,121,600	100.0
Employment status • Unemployed	11	1.6	11	1.6	115,000	3.7
• Employed	416	60.4	408	59.6	1,973,335	63.2
• Not in the labour force	262	38.0	266	38.8	1,033,285	33.1
Total	689	100.0	685	100.0	3,121,620	100.0
Marital status • Now married	406	58.2	395	56.6	1,728,875	54.7
• Live-in partner	72	10.3	70	10.0	276,130	8.8
• Single—never married	72	10.3	95	13.6	653,715	20.7
• Divorced	73	10.5	68	9.8	212,535	6.7
• Separated	19	2.7	20	2.9	92,705	2.9
• Widowed	56	8.0	50	7.1	196,365	6.2
Total	698	100.0	698	100.0	3,160,325	100.0

For the weighted sample, of those respondents who revealed their gender (N = 693), nearly two-thirds (65.9%) were female. Of 690 respondents answering the age question, 44.1% were aged 20–44 and 34.8% were 55 or older, ranging from 18 to 96. Twenty-one percent of 688 respondents held a university degree and another 29.7% held a diploma or certificate from a trade, technical, business or community college. Sixty percent of 685 respondents answering the question were employed full-time and 56.6% of 698 respondents were married, with another 10.0% having a live-in partner.

Comparing the figures for the weighted sample with those of the 2006 census, one finds that the age and education values are practically the same, the weighted sample has 3 percentage points fewer of employed people, 2 percentage points more of married people and 15 percentage points more of females than the census. Since some studies have found women to be generally more supportive than men of the arts (Decima, 2002, p. 50, DiMaggio & Pettitt, 1999, p. 34), the over-representation of women in our sample may create a bias in favour of arts-related activities. In fact, split-file analyses (not shown here) by gender revealed very few differences. If the weighted sample has a bias in favour of arts-related activities, it is a bias shared fairly equally among respondents regardless of their gender, i.e., it is a bias resulting from self-selection of respondents. Gender had no significant impact on any dependent variables in our multiple regression analyses (Sect. "Multivariate Relationships"). In any event, with the exception of gender, our weighted sample is fairly representative of the total population of British Columbia.

Descriptive Statistics

Table 2.2 lists the top 10 arts-related activities by numbers and percent of participants, with average hours per week participation and mean levels of satisfaction. The activity with the highest percentage of participants was listening to music, followed by reading novels, short stories, plays or poetry. Eighty-four percent (593)

Table 2.2 Top 10 arts-related activities by number and percent

Activities	N	%	Hours per week	Mean sat.
Listening to music	593	83.8	14.0	6.0
Reading novels, etc.	412	58.2	7.4	6.1
Watching films, DVD	293	41.4	5.4	5.6
Singing alone	260	36.7	4.3	5.7
Reading to others	216	30.5	3.5	6.0
Telling stories	141	19.9	3.0	5.9
Gourmet cooking	124	17.5	4.6	6.2
Painting or drawing	120	17.0	5.0	5.9
Singing in a group	100	14.1	2.8	6.1
Watching TV art shows	92	13.0	3.7	5.6

reported listening to music an average of 14.0 h per week with a mean level of satisfaction of 6.0. Fifty-eight percent (412) reported reading novels, etc. an average of 7.4 h per week with a mean level of satisfaction of 6.1. The third and fourth activities with the highest percentages of participants were watching of participants, with average number of hours per week participation and mean levels of satisfaction films on DVD or video and singing alone, respectively. Forty-one percent (293) of respondents reported watching films on DVD or video on average 5.4 h per week with a mean level of satisfaction of 5.6. Thirty-seven percent (260) of respondents reported singing alone on average 4.3 h per week with a mean level of satisfaction of 5.7. The activity with the fifth highest percentage of participants was reading to others. Thirty-one percent (216) reported reading to others an average of 3.5 h per week with a mean level of satisfaction of 6.0. Comparing the figures in the first five rows of Table 2.2 with their counterparts in Exhibit 2 of Michalos and Kahlke (2008), one finds the same activities ordered in the same way, practically the same average levels of satisfaction, and a bit more disparity among percentages and hours per week of participation.

Table 2.3 lists the top 10 arts-related activities by numbers and percent of participants, with average times per year participation and mean levels of satisfaction. The activity with the highest percentage of participants was going to films (cinema, movie theatres). Fifty-eight percent (409) reported going to films an average of 6.2 times per year with a mean level of satisfaction of 5.6. The activity with the second highest percentage of participants was going to concerts. Fifty-four percent (384) reported going to concerts an average of 3.5 times per year, with a mean level of satisfaction of 6.0. The activity with the third highest percentage of participants was attending community festivals. Fifty percent (353) of respondents reported attending community festivals an average of 2.9 times per year, with a mean level of satisfaction of 5.6. The activities with the fourth and fifth highest percentages of participants were going to historic, heritage sites and going to art museums and galleries, and the figures were similar. Forty-nine percent (348) reported going to historic, heritage sites an average of 3.0 times per year, with a mean level of

Table 2.3 Top 10 arts-related activities by number and percent of participants, with average number of times per year participation and mean levels of satisfaction

Activities	N	%	Times per year	Mean sat.
Go to movies	409	57.7	6.2	5.6
Go to concerts	384	54.2	3.5	6.0
Go to community festivals	353	49.9	2.9	5.6
Go to historic sites	348	49.2	3.0	5.9
Go to art museums	345	48.7	3.4	5.7
Go to other museums	295	41.6	2.3	5.7
Go to public library	295	41.7	8.2	5.6
Go to amateur theatre	264	37.3	2.4	5.8
Go to prof. theatre	254	35.8	2.7	6.2
Decorating a home	212	29.9	5.9	5.8

satisfaction of 5.9, while 49% (345) reported going to art museums and galleries an average of 3.4 times per year, with a mean level of satisfaction of 5.7. Comparing the figures in the first five rows of Table 2.3 with their counterparts in Exhibit 3 of Michalos and Kahlke (2008), one again finds the same activities ordered in the same way, practically the same average levels of satisfaction, and a bit more disparity among percentages and times per year of participation.

Table 2.4 lists the percent of respondents indicating the first thing they think of when they hear the word 'arts' or the phrase 'artistic activity' and respondents' most important arts-related activity, with mean levels of satisfaction with nine aspects of that activity. The most frequently mentioned activity that respondents think of when they hear the word 'arts' or the phrase 'artistic activity' is painting and/or drawing. Thirty-eight percent of the sample gave that response. The most frequently mentioned 'most important' arts-related activity is music in some form. Thirty-six percent gave that response. The most frequently mentioned place where respondents first learned about their most important arts-related activity is in school. Fifty-five percent gave that response. The mean age at which respondents first learned about their most important arts-related activity was 12.0 years. Mean satisfaction levels reported for respondents' access to information about their most important arts-related activity (5.3), access to the activity itself (5.4), access to the place where the activity occurs (5.0) and about the place itself (5.2) were all on the positive side of the 7-point satisfaction scale. For the remaining five items in the list, three items had mean satisfaction levels in the middle range and two were on the negative side. Mean satisfaction levels reported for the price ($) paid for participating in respondents' most important arts-related activity, for city government support and support from other sources for the activity were 4.8, 4.1 and 4.4, respectively. For the amount of provincial government support and federal government support, the mean satisfaction levels were 3.8 and 3.5, respectively. Comparing the items in Table 2.4 with their counterparts in Exhibit 4 of Michalos and Kahlke (2008), one

Table 2.4 Percent of respondents, age, % and sat

Access to activity itself (N)	5.4 (599)
Access to information re activity (N)	5.3 (616)
Place where activity occurs (N)	5.2 (463)
Access to the activity facility (N)	5.0 (558)
Price ($) for participating (N)	4.8 (479)
City government support for activity (N)	4.1 (501)
Provincial government support (N)	3.8 (481)
Federal government support (N)	3.5 (474)
Other support for the activity (N)	4.4 (455)

again finds the same two activities ordered in the same way, the same age and place of first encounter, and practically the same average levels of satisfaction for all items.

Twenty-three of the 45 statements in our questionnaire about beliefs and feelings about arts-related activities were used to construct four indexes of beliefs and feelings that might motivate people to engage in arts-related activities. Since correlation coefficients cannot identify the direction of causality between significantly related variables, it is possible that significant correlations arise because the experience with arts-related activities leads to certain beliefs and feelings about the activities. Most likely, the causal arrows run in both directions although we are using the general label of 'motivational indexes' for the four. Table 2.5 lists each of the four indexes by name, gives the statements included in each, the percent of respondents agreeing or strongly agreeing with each statement, the item-total correlation of each statement with the index and Cronbach's Alpha Coefficient of Reliability. Each index is formed by simply summing the values of the variables included in it. Besides the four arts-related indexes, Table 2.5 also lists the same information for three overall life assessment indexes.

Table 2.5a describes the Index of Arts as Self-Health Enhancers, which has six items and an Alpha Coefficient of a = 0.87. A good representative item is 'My artistic activities contribute to my emotional wellbeing', which has an item-total correlation of r = 0.80. Eighty-eight percent of respondents agreed or strongly agreed with this statement.

Table 2.5b describes the Index of Arts as Self-Developing Activities, which has six items and an a = 0.86. A good representative item is 'My artistic activities contribute to my self-esteem', which has an item-total correlation of r = 0.71. Seventy-five percent of respondents agreed or strongly agreed with this statement.

Table 2.5c describes the Index of Arts as Community Builders, which has six items and an a = 0.82. A good representative item is 'Artistic activity strengthens a community', which has an item-total correlation of r = 0.61. Seventy-eight percent of respondents agreed or strongly agreed with this statement.

Table 2.5d describes the Index of Arts and Arts-Related Activities as Ends in Themselves, which has five items and an a = 0.71. A good representative item is 'I enjoy art for its own sake', which has an item-total correlation of r = 0.64. Eighty-eight percent of respondents agreed or strongly agreed with this statement.

Table 2.5e describes the Satisfaction With Life Scale (SWLS) developed by Diener et al. (1985), which has five items and an a = 0.90. A good representative item is 'I am satisfied with my life', which has an item-total correlation of r = 0.83. Forty-nine percent of respondents agreed or strongly agreed with this statement.

Table 2.5f describes the Contentment with Life Assessment Scale (CLAS) developed by Lavallee et al. (2007), which has five items and an a = 0.87. A good representative item is 'I am very content with my life', which has an item-total correlation of r = 0.76. Forty eight percent of respondents agreed or strongly agreed with this statement.

Table 2.5 Indexes of beliefs and feelings that might motivate arts-related activity, whole group, satisfaction with life scale (SWLS), contentment with life assessment scale (CLAS) and subjective wellbeing (SWB)

Item	% Agreeing or strongly agreeing	Item-total correlation
a. Index of arts as self-health enhancers, N = 648, a = .87[a] Description: My artistic activities…		
• Have a positive effect on my life	90.0	0.58
• Help me to relax	89.8	0.70
• Help relieve stress	86.0	0.72
• Contribute to my emotional wellbeing	88.0	0.80
• Help me to stay healthy	66.8	0.55
• Contribute to my overall wellbeing	78.8	0.70
b. Index of arts as self-developing activities, N = 642, a = .86[b] Description: My artistic activities…		
• Give me self-confidence	76.1	0.64
• Help me to learn about myself	73.8	0.65
• Help me to reveal my thoughts, feelings or physical skills to others	72.3	0.64
• Contribute to my self-esteem	74.5	0.71
• Help me develop my social skills	59.9	0.53
• Help me express my personal identity	67.4	0.69
c. Index of arts as community builders, N = 637, a = .82[c]		
• My artistic activities help me to learn about other people	74.6	0.55
• My artistic activities help me to accept differences among people	71.4	0.55
• My artistic activities help me feel connected to this community	49.0	0.53
• Artists help build community solidarity	70.2	0.59
• Artistic activity strengthens a community	77.7	0.61
• Artistic activity in a community increases its social capital	62.9	0.62
d. Index of arts and arts-related activities as ends in themselves, N = 639, a = .71[d]		
• The appreciation of art is an art-lover's reward	66.2	0.39
• Good art needs no justification beyond itself	72.5	0.51
• I enjoy art for its own sake	88.3	0.64
• Without art, life would be very dull	84.1	0.42
• I engage in artistic activities for the sake of the activities themselves	68.2	0.38
e. Satisfaction with life scale (SWLS), N = 667, a = .90[e]		
• In most ways my life is close to my ideal	35.3	0.78

(continued)

Table 2.5 (continued)

Item	% Agreeing or strongly agreeing	Item-total correlation
• The conditions of my life are excellent	42.3	0.79
• I am satisfied with my life	49.1	0.83
• So far I have gotten the important things I want out of life	52.6	0.78
• If I could live my life over, I would change nothing	34.5	0.60
f. Contentment with life assessment scale (CLAS), N = 661, a = .87[f]		
• Nothing is currently lacking in my life	32.5	0.71
• I am living my life to the fullest	32.8	0.79
• I am very content with my life	48.1	0.76
• When I examine my life as a whole, I feel that I am not meeting 29.2 my aspirations. (reverse coded)		0.60
• I feel dissatisfied because I'm not doing everything that I want to 28.3 be doing in my life. (reverse coded)		0.64
	% Very or somewhat sat.	**Item-total correlation**
g. Subjective wellbeing (SWB), N = 675, a = 0.87[g]		
• How satisfied are you with Your life as a whole	67.2	0.76
• Your overall standard of living	64.7	0.63
• Your overall quality of life	65.8	0.80
	% Very or somewhat hap.	**Item-total correlation**
• How happy would you say you are?	76.4	0.68

[a] Scale mean = 24.6, standard deviation = 3.7
[b] Scale mean = 22.8, standard deviation = 4.1
[c] Scale mean = 22.5, standard deviation = 3.6
[d] Scale mean = 19.7, standard deviation = 2.9
[e] Scale mean = 24.2, standard deviation = 6.7
[f] Scale mean = 22.2, standard deviation = 6.6
[g] Scale mean = 23.0, standard deviation = 4.1

Table 2.5g describes the Subjective Wellbeing Index (SWB) developed by Michalos et al. (2005), which has four items and an a = 0.87. It is constructed by summing responses to four single-item overall life assessment statements concerning one's satisfaction with life as a whole, overall standard of living and quality of life, and one's happiness. Of the four items in the scale, satisfaction with one's overall quality of life has the highest item-total correlation, r = 0.80.

Table 2.6 lists the mean levels of domain and overall life satisfaction and happiness. Generally speaking, with the 7-point satisfaction scale and sample sizes of about 500, differences between mean scores of 0.3 or fewer percentage points are not statistically significant at the modest level of 0.05%, i.e., 19 times out of 20 one might find such differences appearing merely by chance. Of the34 entries in the

Table 2.6 Number of respondents and mean levels of domain and life assessment satisfaction and happiness

Satisfaction with	N	Mean sat.
Your house, apartment, mobile home	694	5.7
Your neighbourhood	693	5.7
Your city, town or rural area	692	5.6
Your family relations, generally	687	5.7
Your living partner	575	6.1
Your job	572	5.4
Your life as a whole	688	5.8
Your friendships	691	5.7
Your physical health	693	5.1
Your psychological health	690	5.4
Your religion or spiritual fulfilment	658	5.2
Your overall standard of living	693	5.6
Your financial security	691	5.0
Your recreation activities	692	5.1
Your level of physical activity	694	4.6
Your level of social activity	689	4.6
Air quality where you live	693	5.2
Drinking water quality where you live	689	5.5
Land pollution where you live	680	4.8
Your sense of meaning in life	690	5.5
Your self-esteem	690	5.5
Your amount of free time	686	4.9
Local primary and secondary schools	613	4.8
Your personal safety near your home	688	5.6
Federal government officials	676	3.6
Provincial government officials	677	3.6
Local government officials	670	4.0
Your overall quality of life	690	5.7
How local people treat you	692	5.7
Your access to health care	687	5.2
What you achieve in life	689	5.3
Your future security	686	5.1
Feeling part of your community	688	5.0
Your overall happiness	690	5.9

exhibit, 26 (77%) are on the positive side of the 7-point satisfaction and happiness scales. Of the 3 entries concerning satisfaction with government officials, two are the lowest of all the scores in the table. The scores for satisfaction with federal and provincial officials are the same, 3.6, which means a little dissatisfied. Satisfaction with local government officials just reaches the scale mid-point of 4.0. The mean score for satisfaction with one's living partner (6.1) is the highest in the table and the only one in the table above 6.0. Other items with mean scores clustered at the top of the list include overall happiness (5.9) and satisfaction with life as a whole

Table 2.7 Number of respondents and mean scores on respondents' lives compared to diverse standards

Your life now compared to	N	Mean
What you want from life	687	5.5
What others your age and sex have	692	5.1
What you deserve	684	4.6
What you need	686	4.7
What you expected it would be now	687	4.6
What you expect it to be in 5 years	688	4.8
The best in your previous experience	690	4.6

(5.8). Ignoring the scores for government officials, the cluster of items at the bottom of the list include satisfaction with one's level of social and physical activity (each 4.6), local land pollution and primary and secondary schools (each 4.8), and amount of free time (4.9). Comparing the items in Table 2.6 with their counterparts in Exhibit 7 of Michalos and Kahlke (2008), one again finds striking similarities. In the five-communities study, 75% of 204 entries were on the positive side of the 7-point scales, with satisfaction with one's living partner again at the top (6.2), followed by overall happiness (5.9). The three government items were again at the bottom, only none reached the mid-point of the scale. Ignoring the scores for government officials, the cluster of items at the bottom of the list began again with satisfaction with one's level of social and physical activity (each 4.7), local land pollution and primary and secondary schools (each 4.8), and amount of free time and local air quality (each 4.9).

Table 2.7 lists mean scores on respondents' lives compared to seven different self-assessment standards. Mean scores reveal that respondents were on the positive side of two of the seven scales. On average, respondents scored 5.5 on the have-want scale, indicating that all things considered, their lives provided more than half of what they wanted. They also thought that their lives provided more than the lives of the average person of their sex and age in their local area (5.1). This sort of ego-centric bias has been reported by many researchers, e.g., see Michalos (1991), pp. 123–124. Regarding the other 5 standards, their scores were only in the middle range, though on the favourable side. Comparing their lives to what they expect to have in 5 years, they scored 4.8; compared to what they need, they scored 4.7. For the remaining three comparisons, they scored each the same, 4.6. Comparing the items in Table 2.7 with their counterparts in Exhibit 8 of Michalos and Kahlke (2008), one again finds the same two clusters above and below the positive side of the scale, with the same two items at the top in the same order.

Bivariate Relationships

The main task of this section is to review 8 sets of correlational studies to discover connections among all our survey variables that seem to be interesting in themselves, suggestive of other likely relationships and potentially useful for the even more interesting multivariate investigations in the following section.

Table 2.8 lists results of correlating the average number of hours per week engaged in each of 22 arts-related activities and each activity's corresponding mean level of satisfaction (44 items total) with mean scores on our seven overall assessments of life, i.e., self-reported general health (GH), satisfaction with life as a whole (Lsat), happiness with life as a whole (Hap), satisfaction with the overall quality of life (qolsat), satisfaction with life as a whole index (SWLS), contentment with life assessment scale (CLAS), and subjective wellbeing (SWB). As well, the average number of hours per week engaged in each of the arts-related activities is correlated with each activity's corresponding mean level of satisfaction (Act. Sat. in column one of the table). We arbitrarily selected N = 30 as a cut-off figure and examined all zero-order linear associations (Pearson Product Moment Correlations) for activities

Table 2.8 Correlations among average number of hours per week engaged in arts-related activities and levels of satisfaction with each activity (Act.Sat.) and seven life assessment variables: general health (GH), life satisfaction (Lsat), happiness (hap), satisfaction with overall quality of life (qolsat), satisfaction with life scale (SWLS), contentment with life assessment scale (CLAS) and subjective wellbeing (SWB)

Activity	Act.Sat.	GH	Lsat	hap	qolsat	SWLS	CLAS	SWB	NC
Age	–	ns	0.11	0.09	0.09	0.16	0.19	0.15	657
Education	–	0.22	ns	ns	ns	0.09	ns	0.09	654
House/income	–	ns	0.09	0.11	0.16	0.15	0.12	0.19	504
Body Mass Index	–	−0.18	ns	ns	ns	ns	ns	ns	623
Listening/music	0.09	ns	ns	ns	ns	ns	ns	ns	566
Reading novels	0.28	ns	ns	ns	ns	ns	ns	ns	390
Re/nov/sat	1.00	0.12	0.15	0.16	0.12	ns	ns	0.15	390
Watch films DVD	ns	−0.14	ns	ns	ns	ns	ns	ns	281
Singing alone	0.25	ns	−0.12	ns	ns	ns	ns	ns	248
Singing alone sat	1.00	ns	ns	0.21	0.13	ns	0.19	0.14	248
Read to others	0.26	ns	ns	ns	ns	ns	ns	ns	206
Read others sat	1.00	ns	ns	0.19	ns	ns	ns	ns	206
Telling stories	0.22	ns	ns	ns	ns	−0.22	−0.18	ns	135
Tell stories sat	1.00	ns	ns	0.21	ns	ns	ns	ns	135
Gourmet cooking	0.26	ns	ns	ns	ns	ns	ns	ns	115
Gour/cook/sat	1.00	ns	ns	0.36	ns	ns	ns	0.19	115
Painting, drawing	0.25	ns	ns	ns	−0.19	ns	ns	ns	116
Paint/draw/sat	1.00	0.18	ns	0.20	ns	ns	ns	ns	116
Watch TV art	ns	0.33	ns	ns	0.24	ns	ns	ns	87
Watch TV art/sat	1.00	ns	ns	ns	ns	ns	−0.23	ns	87
Play/music/inst.	0.27	ns	ns	−0.26	ns	ns	ns	ns	66
Knit/crochet/sat	1.00	ns	ns	ns	0.30	ns	ns	ns	56
Take/kids/arts	ns	−0.39	ns	ns	ns	ns	ns	ns	51
Take/kids/arts/sat	1.00	ns	−0.34	ns	−0.28	ns	−0.28	−0.31	51
Arranging flowers sat	1.00	ns	ns	0.35	0.36	0.36	0.37	0.34	44
Make clothes sat	1.00	ns	ns	ns	0.39	ns	ns	0.41	35

P\0.05

involving that many respondents or more. The last column in the table gives the minimum sample size involved in each of the correlations for each row. The first four rows of the table give the results of correlating 4 demographic variables (age, education, household income and Body Mass Index) with the seven overall life assessments.

Our review of the results in Table 2.8 will begin with a discussion of correlations between each demographic and life assessment variable. Second, we will consider correlations between the average amount of time invested in each arts-related activity and the average amount of obtained satisfaction from that investment (results in column under Act.Sat.). Third, we will examine correlations between time invested and satisfaction obtained for each arts-related activity, on the one hand, with each of the seven life assessment variables, on the other, taking each of the latter variables one at a time. Finally, we will give special attention to some of the variables for time invested and satisfaction obtained that had a relatively extensive impact on most of the seven life assessment variables.

Twenty-eight (4 9 7) associations between the demographic and life assessment variables were measured, and 16 (57.1%) were found to be statistically significant at the P\0.05 level. (To simplify the discussion, we arbitrarily decided to use a single level of significance throughout the study.) No demographic variable was significantly correlated with every life assessment variable, although age and household income were significantly correlated with 6 of the 7. General Health scores were not correlated with age or household income, which is unusual and inconsistent with results reported in Michalos and Kahlke (2008, Exhibit 9). On average, age was correlated with the 6 life assessment variables at $r = 0.13$, with a high of $r = 0.19$ for the Contentment with Life Assessment Scale (CLAS) and a low of $r = 0.09$ for happiness (Hap) and satisfaction with the overall quality of life (qolsat). Education and the Body Mass Index were significantly correlated with three and one of the seven life assessment variables, respectively. Generally speaking, the 4 demographic variables had weaker associations with the 7 life assessment variables in the British Columbia sample than in the five-communities sample.

Since we began with 22 arts-related activities that had at least 30 people engaged in them and each activity produced its own corresponding mean level of satisfaction, there were 22 9 2 = 44 distinct variables to correlate with 7 life assessment variables, giving a possible 308 significant correlation coefficients. Besides these 308 coefficients, there might have been 22 more indicating significant associations between each arts-related activity and its corresponding mean level of satisfaction. The fact that there are only 22 rows of arts-related activities and/or corresponding satisfaction items in Table 2.8 shows that 22 (50.0%) of the 44 distinct variables had no significant correlations with any of the life assessment variables and/or a corresponding level of satisfaction variable. Considering only the 22 variables listed in Table 2.8, if every measurement had produced a statistically significant result then there would have been 154 (22 9 7) cells with numerical values indicating significant associations between arts-related activities and/or corresponding levels of satisfaction with each of the 7 life assessment variables plus 8 more values indicating significant associations between each activity variable and its corresponding satisfaction variable, rather than the 45 values displayed in the table. Thus, for our sample of 708 respondents, subtracting the 8 values listed in the column headed Act. Sat., there are only 37 cases out of our original possible 308 (12.0%) of the time spent on activities variables and/or variables indicating the satisfaction obtained from those activities that had significant correlations with our 7 life assessment variables. Considering only the 22 variables listed in Table 2.8, there are 37 of 154 (24.0%) cases that had significant correlations with the 7 life assessment variables.

Since a person's engagement in arts-related activities is usually voluntary, one might expect a statistically significant positive correlation between the time spent engaged in arts-related activities and the level of satisfaction obtained from the engagement. Although there are no negative correlations in the Activity Satisfaction (Act.Sat.) column, 3 associations were not statistically significant. However, because the average number of hours per week engaged in 11 of the original 22 arts-related activities did not have statistically significant associations with any other variables, including their corresponding measures of satisfaction, these 11 are not listed in the exhibit. There were, then, a total of 14 (63.6%) activities (3 listed in the table and 11 not listed) with statistically insignificant correlations with their corresponding mean levels of satisfaction. In all these cases, apparently the average satisfaction obtained from participation in arts-related activities cannot be the sole or even primary motivator of engagement. A similar anomaly appears in Table 2.9 regarding arts-related activities with engagement measured in number of times per year, and it was also reported in Michalos and Kahlke (2008) for the corresponding tables (Exhibits 9 and 10).

A casual glance at Table 2.8 suggests that there is a great variety of relationships between the average number of hours per week engaged in arts-related activities and the corresponding mean levels of satisfaction resulting from that engagement, on the one hand, and the seven life assessment variables, on the other. If one tried to measure the impact of arts-related activities on the perceived quality of people's lives using only one of these seven scales as one's dependent variable, one would inevitably underestimate that impact. Nine (41.0%) of the 22 arts-related activities and/or corresponding mean levels of satisfaction resulting from engagement in those activities had a significant correlation with only one life assessment variable, and five (22.7%) more had such a correlation with two life assessment variables.

Close inspection of the seven life assessment columns in Table 2.8 reveals that the satisfaction with life index (SWLS) had the fewest number (2) of significant associations with the average number of hours per week engaged in the 22 arts-related activities and/or the corresponding mean levels of satisfaction resulting from that engagement. Two life assessment variables had 8 significant correlations with the 22 arts-related activities and/or the corresponding mean levels of satisfaction resulting from that engagement, namely, the single-item measure of satisfaction with the overall quality of life (qolsat) and the single-item happiness measure (Hap). On average, for the eight significant correlations with qolsat, $r = 0.13$, and with Hap, $r = 0.18$. Regarding happiness, correlation coefficients ran from a positive high of $r = 0.35$ for the satisfaction obtained from arranging flowers to a negative low of

Table 2.9 Correlations among average number of times per year engaged in arts-related activities and levels of satisfaction with each activity (Act.Sat.) and life assessment variables: general health (GH), life satisfaction (Lsat), happiness (hap), satisfaction with overall quality of life (qolsat), satisfaction with life scale (SWLS), contentment with life assessment scale (CLAS) and subjective wellbeing (SWB)

Activity	Act.Sat.	GH	Lsat	hap	qolsat	SWLS	CLAS	SWB	NC
Go to movies	0.22	ns	ns	ns	ns	ns	−0.12	ns	390
Go concerts	0.15	ns	ns	ns	ns	ns	ns	ns	367
Go concert sat	1.00	ns	0.16	0.17	0.13	ns	ns	0.17	367
Go his/her site	0.15	ns	ns	ns	0.15	0.11	ns	0.14	333
Go his/her sat	1.00	ns	ns	ns	0.14	ns	0.15	0.13	333
Go art museum	0.10	ns	ns	ns	ns	ns	ns	ns	330
Go art museum sat	1.00	0.15	0.20	0.19	0.17	0.16	0.14	0.22	330
Go other museum sat	1.00	0.15	0.23	0.19	0.21	0.22	0.17	0.26	284
Go public library	0.29	ns	ns	ns	ns	ns	ns	ns	283
Go public library sat	1.00	ns	0.14	ns	ns	0.14	ns	ns	283
Go amateur theatre	0.23	0.14	ns	ns	ns	ns	ns	ns	251
Go amateur theatre sat	1.00	0.14	0.34	0.22	0.31	0.32	0.23	0.35	251
Go prof theatre sat	1.00	ns	0.29	0.25	0.23	0.26	0.23	0.29	243
Decorating home	0.14	ns	ns	ns	ns	ns	ns	ns	201
Decorating home sat	1.00	ns	0.15	0.17	ns	ns	ns	ns	201
Go to school plays sat	1.00	ns	0.22	0.23	0.17	0.22	0.18	0.24	204
Buy art work	0.14	ns	ns	ns	ns	ns	ns	ns	198
Buy art work sat	1.00	ns	0.22	0.15	0.24	ns	0.17	0.22	198
Des. Garden sat	1.00	ns	ns	ns	0.15	ns	0.20	ns	187
Go dancing	0.15	ns	ns	ns	ns	ns	ns	ns	173
Go dancing sat	1.00	ns	ns	ns	0.18	ns	ns	ns	173
Wk com. Fes sat	1.00	ns	ns	0.25	ns	ns	ns	ns	90
Give art dona sat	1.00	ns	0.22	ns	ns	0.32	0.29	ns	84
Figure skating	0.33	ns	ns	ns	ns	ns	ns	ns	35
Figure skating sat	1.00	ns	ns	0.39	ns	ns	ns	ns	35

P\0.05

r = −0.26 for the average number of hours per week playing music. Regarding satisfaction with the overall quality of life, correlation coefficients ran from a positive high of r = 0.39 for the satisfaction obtained from making clothes to a negative low of r = −0.28 for the satisfaction obtained from taking children to arts-related activities.

While we were prepared to find that the average amount of time invested in some arts-related activities was negatively associated with one or another life assessment variable (cf. Michalos & Kahlke, 2008, Exhibit 9), we were surprised to find that the average level of satisfaction obtained from engaging in some arts-related activities could have negative associations. Nevertheless, Table 2.8 shows that there were five such cases, involving the satisfaction obtained from watching art shows on television and taking children to arts-related activities. Remarkably, the only statistically significant associations these four arts-related satisfaction variables had with any overall life assessment variables were negative. What's more, neither of the two arts-related satisfaction variables had significant associations with the average number of hours per week invested in the corresponding arts-related activities, e.g., there was no significant correlation between the average number of hours per week spent watching art programs on television and satisfaction obtained from such activity. So, some respondents spent some time engaged in arts-related activities that generated immediate satisfaction that had no significant association with the activities themselves but was significantly and negatively related to some overall life assessment variables. How can we explain engagement in such activities and the negative impact that satisfaction from such engagement has on life assessment variables?

One might argue that one of the two arts-related activities is not a case of engaging in art at all, i.e., driving kids to some kind of artistic event or facility is not engaging in art. So, for present purposes the negative association between satisfaction obtained from such activities and life assessment measures is irrelevant. Unfortunately, this does not address the problem that some kinds of satisfaction have a negative impact on other kinds of satisfaction. It is generally assumed, in the bottom-up explanatory model of perceived life satisfaction for example, that satisfaction from diverse sources and possibly of diverse kinds is routinely combined to produce satisfaction with life as a whole. While it is easy to understand how the time invested in driving one's kids to an art class might have a negative impact on one's life satisfaction (although we have no evidence that it did), it is far from clear why the satisfaction obtained from driving one's kids to the class should have a negative impact. Why should feeling good about driving one's kids to class have a negative impact on how one feels about one's life as a whole? Apparently the activity is some kind of a mixed blessing. One drives the kids to art class feeling pretty good about it because it makes the kids happy and is the right thing to do. Nevertheless, that pretty good feeling is not measurably significantly associated with the activity itself but has the unintended consequence of depressing one's satisfaction with the overall quality of life. The actor performs an act somewhat begrudgingly and the modest level of satisfaction obtained from it takes a heavy negative toll on the actor's overall life assessment.

There clearly are associations between time invested in activities and satisfaction obtained from the investment that were too weak to be captured by some of our measuring instruments, e.g., we have reported satisfaction obtained from arranging flowers, and although it had no significant association with the time invested in the activity, it had significant correlations with several overall life assessment variables. It is theoretically possible that the reported satisfaction obtained from arranging flowers is really an effect of some kind of genetically hard-wired core affect that is somehow (wittingly or unwittingly) connected to the activity of arranging flowers. Davern et al. (2007) and Cummins et al. (2007) made an interesting case for such phenomena, although Moum (2007) and Land (2007) were not persuaded. While there must be some genetic connection to people's experiences and feelings, it is far from clear why one's genes would produce certain effects with some arts-related activities and not others. In any event, at this point we have no good genetically based explanation for the oddities just reported.

Inspection of all the figures in the 22 rows concerning arts-related activities and corresponding levels of satisfaction reveals that there are only two cases in which as many as five significant correlations with life assessment variables appear, namely, for the satisfaction obtained from reading novels, etc. and the satisfaction obtained from arranging flowers. On average, for the five significant correlations with the satisfaction obtained from reading novels, etc., r = 0.14, and with the satisfaction obtained from arranging flowers, r = 0.36. While the flower arrangers got a much bigger average boost than the readers of novels, etc. in their life assessment scores, there may have been as few as only 44 of the former compared to as few as 390 of the latter. Regarding the satisfaction obtained from reading novels, etc., correlation coefficients ran from a high of r = 0.16 for happiness to a low of r = 0.12 for general health and satisfaction with the overall quality of life. Regarding the satisfaction obtained from arranging flowers, correlation coefficients ran from a high of r = 0.37 for the contentment with life assessment scale (CLAS) to a low of r = 0.34 for subjective wellbeing.

Considering the relative number of arts-related activities engaged in fairly frequently and/or their corresponding levels of satisfaction that were significantly correlated with Hap and/or qolsat, it seems that if one were looking for associations between such activities and/or their corresponding satisfaction with the perceived quality of life, one's chances for finding such associations would be maximized by using either of these two measures and minimized by using either SWLS or Lsat. Still, one's best strategy would be to use several dependent variables.

As we found in our earlier study, there was some evidence that producing art was more highly correlated with immediate satisfaction than consuming art. Of the eight variables indicating the average number of hours per week engaged in arts-related activities with significant associations, 5 referred to production (i.e., singing alone, gourmet cooking, painting and drawing, playing a musical instrument and telling stories) and 3 referred to consumption (i.e., listening to music, reading novels, etc., and reading to others). On average, the productive activities correlated at r = 0.25 while the consumptive activities correlated at r = 0.21 with the corresponding immediate satisfaction. In the most extreme case, the average number of hours per week engaged in listening to music had a correlation of r = 0.09 with its corresponding satisfaction, compared to the correlation of r = 0.27 between playing a musical instrument and its corresponding satisfaction. Of course, many more respondents could listen to music (at least 566) than produce it (possibly as few as 66).

Table 2.9 lists results of correlating the average number of times per year engaged in each of 19 arts-related activities and each activity's corresponding mean level of satisfaction (38 items total) with mean scores on our 7 overall assessments of life, and correlating the average number of times per year engaged in each of the 19 activities with each activity's corresponding mean level of satisfaction (Act.Sat.). Our cut-off figure for measuring associations was N = 32 simply because the activity with the next lowest number of participants had only N = 8. Our review of the results in this table will follow the pattern established for Table 2.8.

Beginning with 19 arts-related activities that had at least 32 respondents engaged in them and each activity's corresponding mean level of satisfaction, there were 19 9 2 = 38 distinct variables to correlate with 7 life assessment variables, giving a possible 266 significant correlation coefficients. Besides these 266 coefficients, there might have been 19 more indicating significant associations between each arts-related activity and its corresponding mean level of satisfaction. The fact that there are only 25 rows of arts-related activities and/or corresponding satisfaction items in Table 2.9 shows that 13 (34.2%) of the 38 distinct variables had no significant correlations with any of the life assessment variables and/or a corresponding level of satisfaction variable. Considering only the 25 variables listed in Table 2.9, if every measurement had produced a statistically significant result then there would have been 175 (25 9 7) cells with numerical values indicating significant associations between arts-related activities and/or corresponding levels of satisfaction with each of the 7 life assessment variables plus 10 more values indicating significant associations between each activity variable in the table and its corresponding satisfaction variable, rather than the 72 values displayed in the table. Thus, for our sample of 708 respondents, subtracting the 10 values listed in the column headed Act.Sat., there are only 62 cases out of our original possible 175 (35.4%) time spent on activities variables and/or variables indicating the satisfaction obtained from those activities that had significant correlations with our 7 life assessment variables. Although this is not a particularly high percentage, it is larger than that concerning arts-related activities with frequency of participation counted in hours per week. What is perhaps even more interesting is the fact that there is only one negative correlation in Table 2.9. In our earlier study, we found that all the time spent on and the satisfaction obtained from the arts-related activities listed in the times per year table made a positive contribution to one or more of the overall life assessments. Here we find that only the time invested in going to movies has a negative association with one overall life assessment index, i.e., for CLAS, $r = -0.12$.

There are 10 out of a possible 19 (52.6%) statistically significant correlations in the Act.Sat. column, with an average value of $r = 0.19$, ranging from a high of $r = 0.33$ for the average number of times per year respondents engaged in figure skating (How Canadian!) to a low of $r = 0.10$ for the average number of times per year respondents went to art museums. Of course, many more people reported going to art museums (at least 330) than engaging in figure skating (perhaps as few as 35). There is again (as in Table 2.8) a great variety of relationships (i.e., heterogeneity of effects) between the average number of times per year engaged in the 19 arts-related activities and the corresponding mean levels of satisfaction resulting from that engagement, on the one hand, and the 7 life assessment variables, on the other.

Inspection of the 7 life assessment columns in Table 2.9 reveals that General Health (GH) had the fewest number of significant associations with the average number of times per year engaged in the 19 arts-related activities and the corresponding mean levels of satisfaction resulting from that engagement. Three of the 4 correlations with GH are with activity satisfaction variables that have significant and positive associations with each of the 7 life assessment variables. On average, the mean level of satisfaction obtained from visiting art museums has a correlation of r = 0.18 with the 7 life assessment variables, ranging from a high of r = 0.22 for subjective wellbeing (SWB) to a low of r = 0.14 for CLAS. The mean level of satisfaction obtained from visiting other museums has an average correlation of r = 0.20 with the 7 life assessment variables, ranging from a high of r = 0.26 for SWB to a low of r = 0.15 for GH. The mean level of satisfaction obtained from going to amateur theatre performances has an average correlation of r = 0.27 with the 7 life assessment variables, ranging from a high of r = 0.35 for SWB to a low of r = 0.14 for GH.

Satisfaction with the overall quality of life (qolsat) had the largest number of significant and positive associations with the average number of times per year engaged in the 19 arts-related activities and the corresponding mean levels of satisfaction resulting from that engagement. The 11 significant correlations in the qolsat column have an average of r = 0.19, with a high of r = 0.31 for the satisfaction obtained from going to amateur theatre performances to a low of r = 0.13 for the satisfaction obtained from going to concerts. In our earlier study, General Health had the largest number of significant and positive associations with times per year and corresponding satisfaction variables.

Considering the facts that the average level of satisfaction obtained from going to live amateur, professional and school theatre performances are significantly and positively correlated with 7, 6 and 6 of the life assessment variables, respectively, such theatre performances should be given special recognition. As we discovered and emphasized in our earlier study, among the 19 arts-related activities in which people participate relatively infrequently (i.e., participation is counted in times per year rather than in hours per week), live theatre is supreme in the strength of its correlation with respondents' perceived quality of life measured in diverse ways. If this is any reflection of the contribution of dramatists to the quality of human existence for over 2500 years, they may be justifiably proud of it.

Table 2.10 lists results of correlating our 7 life assessment variables with 21 domain satisfaction variables. Three of the domain satisfaction variables are combinations of some of those listed in Table 2.6. Values for the health satisfaction variable appearing in Table 2.10 were obtained by calculating the mean of the scores on the physical and psychological health satisfaction variables. Similarly, values for the environmental satisfaction variable appearing in Table 2.10 were obtained by calculating the mean of the scores on the air, water and land quality satisfaction variables, and values for the government satisfaction variable were obtained by calculating the mean of the scores on the federal, provincial and local government officials satisfaction variables. All of the 147 correlations listed in this table are significant and positive. In the corresponding table of Michalos and Kahlke (2008, Exhibit 11), all of the correlation coefficients are also positive and significant. Examination of the mean values of each row in the table reveals that on average for our respondents, satisfaction with one's health (mean r = 0.60), self-esteem (mean r = 0.59) and the sense of meaning in life (mean r = 0.55) have the largest correlations with the 7 life assessment variables. These were also the top three in our earlier study, with the same order and similar correlation coefficients, i.e., r = 0.64, r = 0.57 and r = 0.54, respectively. Smallest correlations on average were for satisfaction

Table 2.10 Correlations of domain satisfaction scores with life assessment variables: general health (GH), life satisfaction (Lsat), happiness (hap), satisfaction with overall quality of life (qolsat), satisfaction with life scale (SWLS), contentment with life assessment scale (CLAS) and subjective wellbeing (SWB)

Domain sat with	GH	Lsat	hap	qolsat	SWLS	CLAS	SWB	Mean
Your house, apartment	0.11	0.43	0.38	0.44	0.39	0.38	0.51	0.38
Neighbourhood	0.12	0.36	0.34	0.41	0.37	0.32	0.47	0.34
City, town or rural area	0.11	0.34	0.28	0.38	0.33	0.30	0.40	0.31
Family relations	0.11	0.46	0.37	0.41	0.40	0.33	0.49	0.37
Living partner	0.18	0.46	0.37	0.44	0.43	0.32	0.49	0.38
Job	0.20	0.53	0.37	0.40	0.46	0.43	0.51	0.41
Friendships	0.25	0.59	0.47	0.53	0.43	0.43	0.60	0.47
Health	0.63	0.66	0.51	0.62	0.56	0.53	0.68	0.60
Religion/spirit fulfil	0.26	0.43	0.34	0.44	0.43	0.40	0.47	0.40
Financial security	0.25	0.44	0.44	0.55	0.48	0.46	0.64	0.47
Recreation activities	0.39	0.49	0.45	0.60	0.46	0.43	0.61	0.49
Environment	0.18	0.28	0.27	0.37	0.28	0.25	0.36	0.28
Sense of meaning in life	0.23	0.65	0.54	0.61	0.58	0.57	0.68	0.55
Self-esteem	0.29	0.66	0.63	0.63	0.61	0.63	0.71	0.59
Amount of free time	ns	0.35	0.32	0.40	0.32	0.33	0.39	0.35
Personal safety by home	0.19	0.41	0.35	0.50	0.38	0.31	0.50	0.38
Government officials	0.11	0.18	0.15	0.29	0.19	0.21	0.24	0.20
How locals treat you	0.25	0.56	0.44	0.63	0.50	0.48	0.64	0.50
Access to health care	0.21	0.27	0.26	0.38	0.32	0.24	0.36	0.29
Future security	0.25	0.50	0.51	0.62	0.54	0.54	0.67	0.52
Feel part of your comm.	0.19	0.54	0.49	0.58	0.54	0.51	0.63	0.50

N C 553; P\0.05

with government officials (mean r = 0.20), access to health care (mean r = 0.29) and the environment (mean r = 0.28).

Table 2.11 lists the correlations among the 7 life assessment variables, all of which are significant and positive as expected. On average and as usual, General Health (GH) has the lowest levels of association with the others, indicating that respondents recognize important differences between having good health and having a good life, generally speaking. Because happiness (Hap), satisfaction with life as a whole (Lsat) and satisfaction with the overall quality of life (qolsat) are constituents of subjective wellbeing (SWB), the former three variables have on average the highest levels of association with the latter. Considering the facts that (1) respondents recognize a difference between good health and a good life, and (2) qolsat had the greatest number of significant correlations with arts-related activities involving infrequent engagement and tied with Hap for having the greatest number of significant correlations with arts-related activities involving frequent engagement, it seems fair to say that if one were looking for associations between such activities and the perceived quality of life, and if one could only have a single dependent variable, then one's chances for finding such associations would be maximized by using qolsat as that single variable.

Table 2.11 Correlations among seven life assessment variables: general health (GH), life satisfaction (Lsat), happiness (hap), satisfaction with overall quality of life (qolsat), satisfaction with life scale (SWLS), contentment with life assessment scale (CLAS) and subjective wellbeing (SWB)

Variable	GH	Lsat	hap	qolsat	SWLS	CLAS
GH	1.00					
Lsat	0.38	1.00				
Hap	0.32	0.67	1.00			
Qolsat	0.40	0.72	0.64	1.00		
SWLS	0.40	0.68	0.68	0.66	1.00	
CLAS	0.31	0.64	0.66	0.61	0.80	1.00
SWB	0.41	0.87	0.83	0.88	0.76	0.72

N C 639; P\0.05

Table 2.12 Correlations among average number of hours per week engaged in arts-related activities and levels of satisfaction with motivational indexes: index of arts as self-health enhancers (Health), index of arts as self-developing activities (S-Dev), index of arts as community builders (Comb), index of arts as ends in themselves (Ends) and demographics

Activity	Health	S-Dev	Comb	Ends	NC
Age	−0.08	−0.11	ns	ns	629
Education	0.16	0.09	0.15	0.13	628
Body Mass Index	−0.22	−0.21	−0.21	−0.14	604
Listening to music	0.10	0.13	ns	0.13	545
Listening to music satisfaction	0.28	0.24	0.17	0.22	545
Reading novels satisfaction	ns	0.12	0.15	ns	380
Singing alone satisfaction	0.32	0.33	0.15	0.16	249
Reading to others satisfaction	0.25	ns	ns	ns	206
Gourmet cooking	ns	ns	ns	−0.20	117
Gourmet cooking satisfaction	0.25	ns	ns	ns	117
Painting or drawing	ns	ns	ns	0.25	113
Painting or drawing satisfaction	0.27	0.24	ns	0.20	113
Singing in a group satisfaction	0.26	ns	ns	ns	91
Watching TV art satisfaction	0.24	ns	ns	ns	84
Playing musical instrument sat.	0.33	ns	0.31	ns	64
Arranging flowers	ns	ns	ns	0.33	43
Arranging flowers satisfaction	0.37	0.40	ns	ns	43
Writing novels…etc. sat.	ns	0.48	ns	ns	30
Making clothes	ns	ns	ns	0.53	35
Teaching painting/drawing sat.	ns	ns	0.37	ns	29

P\0.05

Tables 2.12 and 2.13 display results of measuring associations among our four indexes that might provide motives for people engaging in arts-related activities, might summarize beliefs and feelings that arise as effects of experiences with arts-related activities or, as suggested earlier, most likely both. We will need longitudinal studies with panels of participants in order to properly assess these issues. Our review of these two tables will be parallel to our reviews of Tables 2.8 and 2.9, with Table 2.12 involving engagement in arts-related activities measured in hours per week and Table 2.13 involving engagement in arts-related activities measured in times per year.

Table 2.12 lists results of correlating the average number of hours per week engaged in each of 22 arts-related activities and each activity's corresponding mean level of satisfaction (44 items total) with mean scores on our four motivational indexes. The fact that there are only 17 rows of arts-related activities and/or corresponding satisfaction items in Table 2.12 shows that 27 (61%) of the 44 distinct variables had no significant correlations with any of the motivational indexes. For this table, 16 associations between the 4 demographic variables and 4 motivational indexes were also measured, and 10 (62.5%) were found to be statistically significant at the P\0.05 level. Household income does not appear in the table because it did not have any significant correlations with the four motivational indexes. Education and the Body Mass Index were significantly correlated with each index,

Table 2.13 Correlations among average number of times per year engaged in arts-related activities and levels of satisfaction with motivational indexes: index of arts as self-health enhancers (Health), index of arts as self-developing activities (S-Dev), index of arts as community builders (Comb), index of arts as ends in themselves (Ends)

Activity	Health	S-Dev	Comb	Ends	NC
Going to movies	ns	0.14	0.13	0.12	384
Going to movies satisfaction	0.11	0.10	ns	0.16	384
Going to concerts	0.12	0.17	0.17	0.15	358
Going to concerts satisfaction	0.16	0.13	0.18	0.19	358
Attending community festivals	0.12	0.16	ns	ns	330
Attending community festivals sat	0.16	0.19	0.20	0.12	330
Visiting historic, heritage sites	ns	0.12	ns	ns	333
Visiting historic, heritage site sat	0.15	0.15	ns	0.13	333
Going to art museums, galleries	0.13	0.16	ns	ns	324
Go…art museums, galleries sat	0.23	0.22	0.26	0.20	324
Go…other museums	0.15	ns	ns	ns	282
Go…other museums sat	0.22	0.19	0.24	0.13	282
Visiting public library sat	0.14	ns	ns	ns	280
Go…amateur live theatre	ns	0.22	0.16	ns	245
Go…amateur live theatre sat	ns	0.13	0.26	ns	245
Go…prof. live theatre sat	0.14	ns	ns	0.16	234
Decorating a home sat	0.23	0.17	ns	ns	200
Volunteering in the arts sat	ns	ns	0.46	ns	200
Go to school plays satisfaction	0.15	0.16	0.27	ns	198
Buying works of art sat	0.17	ns	ns	0.18	200
Designing a garden sat	0.23	ns	ns	ns	188
Making donations to arts sat	0.22	ns	ns	ns	82

P\0.05

positively with an average of r = 0.13 for the former and negatively with an average of r = −0.20 for the latter. Age was negatively correlated with 2 of the 4 indexes, averaging r = −0.10. Thus, for example, believing and/or feeling that engagement in arts-related activities make a positive contribution to one's health is significantly negatively correlated with age (r = −0.08) and Body Mass Index (r = −0.22), and positively correlated with education (r = 0.16). So, as respondents' age and BMI increased, the strength of their avowal of such beliefs and/or feelings decreased, and as their achieved level of education increased, the strength of their avowal of such beliefs and/or feelings increased, and vice versa.

Considering only the 17 non-demographic variables listed in Table 2.12, if every measurement had produced a statistically significant result, then there would have been 68 (4 9 17) cells with numerical values, rather than the 30 values displayed in the table. Thus, only 44% of the time spent on activities variables and/or variables indicating the satisfaction obtained from those activities had significant correlations with our 4 motivational indexes. (There is no comparable figure from the earlier study because the number and composition of arts-related variables and motivational indexes are different.) Inspection of the 4 motivational index columns in this table reveals that the Index of Arts as Community Builders (Comb) had the fewest number of significant associations with the average number of hours per week engaged in the 17 arts-related activities and the corresponding mean levels of satisfaction resulting from that engagement. The 5 significant correlations in the column have an average of r = 0.23, with a high of r = 0.37 for the satisfaction obtained from teaching painting or drawing to a low of r = 0.15 for the satisfaction obtained from reading novels, etc. and singing alone. The Index of Arts as Self-Health Enhancers (Health) had the largest number of significant associations with the average number of hours per week engaged in the 17 arts-related activities and the corresponding mean levels of satisfaction resulting from that engagement. The 10 significant correlations in the Health column have an average of r = 0.27, with a high of r = 0.37 for the satisfaction obtained from arranging flowers to a low of r = 0.10 for the average number of hours per week spent listening to music.

Two arts-related variables in Table 2.12 had significant and positive associations with each of the 4 motivational indexes, and 2 had significant and positive associations with 3 of the 4. Satisfaction obtained from singing alone had an average correlation of r = 0.24 with the 4 motivational indexes, with a high of r = 0.33 for S-Dev and a low of r = 0.15 for Comb. Thus, for example, as respondents' average levels of satisfaction obtained from singing alone increased, the strength of their beliefs and/or feelings that arts-related activities contributed to their health, self-development, and community building, and were also enjoyed as ends in themselves, increased. Satisfaction obtained from listening to music had an average correlation of r = 0.23 with 4 motivational indexes, with a high of r = 0.28 for Health and a low of r = 0.17 for Comb. Satisfaction obtained from painting or drawing had an average correlation of r = 0.24 with 3 of the 4 motivational indexes (missing Comb), with a high of r = 0.27 for Health and a low of r = 0.20 for Ends. Average number of hours per week engaged in listening to music had an average correlation of r = 0.12 with 3 of the 4 motivational indexes (again missing Comb), with a high of r = 0.13 for S-Dev and Ends, and a low of r = 0.10 for Health.

Table 2.13 lists results of correlating the average number of times per year engaged in each of 19 arts-related activities and each activity's corresponding mean level of satisfaction with mean scores on our four motivational indexes (38 items total). If every measurement for Table 2.13 had produced a statistically significant result, then there would have been 152 (4 9 38) cells with numerical values, rather than the 52 values displayed in the exhibit. Thus, for our sample of 708 respondents, 52 of 152 (34.2%) time spent on activities variables and/or variables indicating the satisfaction obtained from those activities had significant correlations with our four motivational indexes. One should notice first that there are no negative correlations in Table 2.13. Whether the causal arrows running from the time spent on the 19 kinds of arts-related activities and the satisfaction obtained from the engagement to beliefs and/or feelings about the arts are stronger, the same, or weaker than the arrows running in the opposite direction, if there is any influence at all, it is positive.

Inspection of the four motivational index columns in Table 2.13 reveals that the Indexes of Arts as Community Builders (Comb) and as Ends in Themselves (Ends) had the fewest number of significant associations (10) with the average number of times per year engaged in the 19 arts-related activities and the corresponding mean levels of satisfaction resulting from that engagement. The Index of Arts as Self-Health Enhancers (Health) had the largest number of significant associations (17) with the average number of times per year engaged in the 19 arts-related activities and the corresponding mean levels of satisfaction resulting from that engagement. The 17 significant correlations in the Health column have an average of r = 0.17, with a high of r = 0.23 for the satisfaction obtained from going to art museums, decorating a home and designing a garden to a low of r = 0.11 for the satisfaction obtained from going to movies.

Five arts-related time-engaged or satisfaction variables had significant correlations with all four motivational variables, and 4 more of the former had such correlations with 3 of the latter 4. First among the five, satisfaction obtained from going to art museums had an average of r = 0.23 for the 4 motivational indexes, with a high of r = 0.26 for Comb and a low of r = 0.20 for Ends. Satisfaction obtained from going to other kinds of museums ran second, with an average of r = 0.20 for the 4 motivational indexes, a high of r = 0.24 for Comb and a low of r = 0.13 for Ends. First among the 3 out of 4 group, satisfaction obtained from going to school plays had an average of r = 0.19 for Health, S-Dev and Comb.

Table 2.14 lists the correlations among the 4 motivational indexes themselves and Table 2.15 lists the correlations among these 4 indexes and our 7 life assessment variables. The four motivational indexes in Table 2.14 are fairly strongly related, with the lowest coefficient at r = 0.53 between Ends, S-Dev and Comb. The Index of Arts as Community Builders was modestly significantly correlated with 6 of the 7 life assessment variables at r = 0.15, with a high of r = 0.24 for General Health and a low of r = 0.09 for happiness (Table 2.15). General Health (GH) was the only life assessment variable significantly associated with all 4 motivational indexes.

Table 2.14 Correlations among motivational indexes: Index of Arts as Self-Health Enhancers (Health), Index of Arts as Self-Developing Activities (S-Dev), Index of Arts as Community Builders (Comb), Index of Arts as Ends in Themselves (Ends)

Index	Health	S-Dev	Comb
Health	1.00		
S-Dev	0.73	1.00	
Comb	0.57	0.65	1.00
Ends	0.59	0.53	0.53

N C 618; P\0.05

Table 2.15 Correlations among motivational indexes and seven life assessment variables

Index	GH	Lsat	hap	qolsat	SWLS	CLAS	SWB
Health	0.21	ns	0.10	0.08	0.08	ns	ns
S-Dev	0.17	ns	0.08	ns	ns	ns	ns
Comb	0.24	0.14	0.09	0.14	0.13	ns	0.13
Ends	0.17	0.09	ns	ns	ns	ns	ns

N C 614; P\0.05

Multivariate Relationships

Stepwise multiple regression was applied to explain the variation in scores for our 7 overall life assessment variables, and each of the next 7 tables (16–22) is laid out in the same format, with three exceptions in which one or two columns were omitted for lack of significant entries. When all columns are included, the left-hand column lists the names of the predictors. Then there is a column headed 'Demog.' containing the standardized regression coefficients (beta values) resulting from regressing a life assessment (dependent) variable on the four demographic (explanatory, predictor or independent) variables. Standardized regression coefficients have means of zero and standard deviations of one, making comparisons of their relative influence on dependent variables easy to discern. Because standardization is sensitive to the particular variance of the variables employed in any sample, one cannot infer that relationships appearing in one sample must appear in others. The second column of figures is headed 'Mot. Index' and it contains the Beta values resulting from regressing the same life assessment variable on our four motivational indexes. The third column of figures is headed 'Hrs/act.sat.' and it contains the results of regressing the same life assessment variable on the set of hours-spent and satisfaction-obtained variables from Table 2.8 that had statistically significant correlations with that life assessment variable. The fourth column of figures is headed 'Times/sat.' and it contains the results of regressing the same life assessment variable on the set of times-spent and satisfaction-obtained variables from Table 2.9 that had statistically significant correlations with that life assessment variable. The fifth column of figures is headed 'Domain sat.' and it contains the results of regressing the same life assessment variable on the 8 variables indicating satisfaction obtained from some domain or aspect of life listed in Table 2.10 that had the largest correlation coefficients with that life assessment variable. Finally, the sixth column of figures is headed 'All Pred' and it contains the results of regressing the same life assessment variable on all of the predictors that achieved statistical significance in the previous five regressions. Because the introduction of any arts-related additional predictors to the set of significant domain satisfaction predictors drastically reduced the sample size (N) for the regression equation, instead of introducing these variables all together, each one was introduced separately. If it achieved statistical significance, it was maintained while the next variable was introduced and if not, it was dropped.

A quick inspection of the seven tables reveals that only two arts-related predictors achieved statistical significance in a final regression equation and only in the regression involving General Health. As well, only one demographic variable achieved statistical significance in a final equation and that was also in the regression involving General Health. This was somewhat similar to the regression results reported in Michalos and Kahlke (2008). In the latter study only the Indexes of Arts as Self-Health Enhancers and Spirit-Building (not used in this study) achieved statistical significance in the final equation of one life assessment variable, namely, satisfaction with the overall quality of life (qolsat). In that study, on five occasions some demographic variable achieved statistical significance.

The first column of figures in Table 2.16 shows that two of our four demographic predictors remained statistically significant when pressed into service together and that collectively they explained 8.0% of the variation in self-reported General Health (GH) scores. The most influential was education, with a Beta value of b = 0.25, followed by the Body Mass Index at b = −0.14. Thus, figuratively speaking, for example, one could say that on average, for every increase of a full unit step (i.e., one standard deviation unit) of education, respondents got an increase of 25.0% of a step in self-reported General Health, with the values of all other predictors held constant. The second column of figures shows that when the four motivational indexes were used together as predictors, two remained statistically significant and they explained

Table 2.16 Regressions of General Health on demographics, motivation indexes, hours/times engaged and satisfaction obtained from arts-related activities and domain satisfaction

Dependent variables	Demog.	Mot.Index	Hours/act.sat.	Domain sat.	All Pred
N	507	596	199	678	241
% of variance expl	8	7	4	17	20
Predictors	b	b	b	b	b
Education	0.25	*	*	*	**
Body Mass Index	−0.14	*	*	*	−0.13
Comm. Building Ind	*	0.19	*	*	0.14
Health enhance Ind.	*	0.10	*	*	**
Watching films DVD	*	*	−0.17	*	−0.13
Reading novels sat.	*	*	0.14	*	**
Recreat act. sat.	*	*	*	0.33	0.25
Self-Esteem sat.	*	*	*	0.15	0.19

* Not in equation, ** significance level too low to enter equation

7.0% of the variance in General Health scores. The Index of Arts as Community Builders (Comb) was most influential, with a Beta value of b = 0.19. The third column of figures shows that two arts-related variables from the hours per week set of predictors remained statistically significant and explained 4.0% of the variance in General Health scores, with the mean level of satisfaction obtained from watching DVD films having the most influence at b = −0.17. The fourth column of figures shows that two of the domain satisfaction predictors remained statistically significant and together they explained 17.0% of the variance in General Health scores. (Because the dependent variable for this table is self-reported General Health and such reports are highly correlated with satisfaction with one's own health (Michalos, 2004), the latter variable was not used as a predictor of General Health.) Reported satisfaction with respondents' recreational activities was most influential, with a b = 0.33, followed by satisfaction with respondents' own self-esteem, b = 0.15. In the final column, we see that five predictors combined to explain 20.0% of the variance in General Health scores (N = 241), with satisfaction with respondents' recreation activity appearing most influential (b = 0.25), followed by self-esteem satisfaction (b = 0.19). Two arts-related predictors remained statistically significant in the last regression. The Index of Arts as Community Builders (Comb) had a b = 0.14 and the average number of hours per week spent watching DVD films had a b = −0.13. In Michalos and Kahlke (2008) we were able to explain 32.0% of the variance in GH scores, with satisfaction with respondents' recreational activities most influential (b = 0.28).

The first column of figures in Table 2.17 shows that only one of our four demographic predictors remained statistically significant and it explained 1.0% of the variation in satisfaction with life as a whole (Lsat) scores. Household income had a Beta value of b = 0.09. The second column of figures shows that one of the 4

Table 2.17 Regressions of life satisfaction on demographics, motivation indexes, hours/times engaged and satisfaction obtained from arts-related activities and domain satisfaction

Dependent variables	Demog.	Mot. Index	Hours/act.sat.	Times/sat.	Domain sat.	All Pred
N	500	593	430	223	550	550
% of variance expl	1	2	3	7	66	66
Predictors	b	b	b	b	b	b
Household income	0.09	*	*	*	*	**
Comm. Building Ind	*	0.15	*	*	*	**
Reading novels sat.	*	*	0.18	*	*	**
Go other museums sat.	*	*	*	0.16	*	**
Go concert sat.	*	*	*	0.16	*	**
Future security sat.	*	*	*	*	0.10	0.10
Job sat.	*	*	*	*	0.20	0.20
Friendship sat	*	*	*	*	0.21	0.21
Health satisfaction	*	*	*	*	0.25	0.25
Sense/mean life sat.	*	*	*	*	0.16	0.16
Self-esteem sat.	*	*	*	*	0.15	0.15

* Not in equation, ** significance level too low to enter equation

motivational indexes remained statistically significant when the 4 were used together and that by itself that one explained only 2.0% of the variance in life satisfaction scores, with the Index of Arts as Community Builders (Comb) having a Beta value of b = 0.15. The third column of figures shows that one arts-related variable from the hours per week set of predictors remained statistically significant and explained 3.0% of the variance in life satisfaction (Lsat) scores. Respondents' mean levels of satisfaction obtained from reading novels, etc. had a b = 0.18. The fourth column of figures shows that two arts-related variables from the times per year set of predictors remained statistically significant. Satisfaction obtained from going to concerts and non-art museums each had a b = 0.16, and together explained 7.0% of the variance in life satisfaction scores. The fifth column of figures shows that six of the domain satisfaction predictors remained statistically significant and together they explained 66.0% of the variance in life satisfaction scores. The most influential explanatory variable was satisfaction with one's own health (b = 0.25), followed by satisfaction with respondents' friendships (b = 0.21). The final column shows that the addition of each of the demographic and arts-related predictors (one at a time with replacement) to the six significant domain satisfaction predictors from the fifth column produced no change in our explanatory power. All the figures in columns five and six are the same, but the 5 double asterisks in the sixth column mean that in the presence of the 6 domain satisfaction predictors, no explanatory power was added by the demographic and arts-related predictors. In our earlier study, we were able to explain 71.0% of the variance in Lsat scores, with satisfaction with one's own health again most influential, (b = 0.24).

The first column of figures in Table 2.18 shows that one demographic predictor remained statistically significant and it explained 1.0% of the variation in happiness (Hap) scores. Household income had a b = 0.12. The second column of figures shows that when the four motivational indexes were used together as predictors, only one remained statistically significant and by itself explained 1.0% of the variance in happiness scores. The Index of Arts as Self-Health Enhancers had a b = 0.11. The third column of figures shows that a single arts-related variable from the hours per week set of predictors remained statistically significant and it explained 2.0% of the variance in happiness scores, with the mean level of satisfaction obtained from singing alone having a b = 0.15. (Notice, then, that while the average number of hours per week invested in singing alone decreased respondents' satisfaction with life as a whole (Table 2.8), the mean level of satisfaction obtained from singing alone increased their happiness (Tables 2.8 and 2.18)). The fourth column of figures shows that one arts-related variable from the times per year set of predictors remained statistically significant. The satisfaction obtained from going to art museums (b = 0.19) explained 3.0% of the variance in happiness scores. The fifth column of figures shows that 5 of the domain satisfaction variables remained statistically significant and explained 45.0% of the variance in happiness scores. The most influential explanatory variable was satisfaction with respondents' own self-esteem, b = 0.35, followed by satisfaction with their future security, b = 0.18. Again, the final column shows that the addition of each of the demographic and arts-related

Table 2.18 Regressions of happiness on demographics, motivation indexes, hours/times engaged and satisfaction obtained from arts-related activities and domain satisfaction

Dependent variables	Demog.	Mot. Index	Hours/act.sat	Times/sat.	Domain sat.	All Pred
N	505	595	235	378	669	669
% of variance expl	1	1	2	3	45	45
Predictors	b	b	b	b	b	b
Household income	0.12	*	*	*	*	**
Health enhance Ind.	*	0.11	*	*	*	**
Singing alone sat.	*	*	0.15	*	*	**
Go art museum sat.	*	*	*	0.19	*	**
Future security sat.	*	*	*	*	0.18	0.18
Recreation act. Sat.	*	*	*	*	0.10	0.10
Friendships sat.	*	*	*	*	0.10	0.10
Health sat.	*	*	*	*	0.10	0.10
Self-esteem sat.	*	*	*	*	0.35	0.35

* Not in equation, ** significance level too low to enter equation

predictors (one at a time with replacement) to the 5 significant domain satisfaction predictors from the fifth column produced no change in our explanatory power. In our earlier study, we were able to explain 51.0% of the variance in Hap scores, with satisfaction with one's own health most influential, b = 0.33.

The first column of figures in Table 2.19 shows that one of our four demographic variables remained statistically significant and explained 2.0% of the variation in satisfaction with the overall quality of life (qolsat) scores. Household income had a b = 0.16. The second column of figures shows that one of the four motivational indexes remained statistically significant and explained 2.0% of the variance in satisfaction with the overall quality of life scores, i.e., the Index of Arts as Community Builders, b = 0.14. The third column of figures shows that a single arts-related variable from the hours per week set of predictors remained statistically significant, satisfaction obtained from singing alone, b = 0.13, and it explained 1.0% of the variance in satisfaction with the overall quality of life scores. The fourth column of figures shows that a single arts-related variable from the times per year set of predictors remained statistically significant, satisfaction obtained from going to historical sites, b = 0.19, and it explained 3.0% of the variance in satisfaction with the overall quality of life scores. The fifth column of figures shows that 7 of the domain satisfaction predictors remained statistically significant and together they explained 60.0% of the variance in satisfaction with the overall quality of life scores. The most influential explanatory variables were satisfaction with respondents' treatment by local residents, b = 0.22, followed by satisfaction with respondents' health, b = 0.19. Again, the final column shows that the addition of each of the demographic and arts-related predictors to the 7 significant domain satisfaction predictors from the fifth column produced no change in our explanatory power. In our earlier study, we were able to explain 63.0% of the variance in qolsat scores, with satisfaction with

Table 2.19 Regressions of satisfaction with the overall quality of life on demographics, motivation indexes, hours/times engaged and satisfaction obtained from arts-related activities and domain satisfaction

Dependent variables	Demog.	Mot. Index	Hours/act.sat.	Times/sat.	Domain sat.	All Pred
N	504	596	236	361	664	664
% of variance expl	2	2	1	3	60	60
Predictors	b	b	b	b	b	b
Household income	0.16	*	*	*	*	**
Comm. Building Ind	*	0.14	*	*	*	**
Singing alone sat.	*	*	0.13	*	*	**
Go historic sites sat.	*	*	*	0.19	*	**
Local treatment sat.	*	*	*	*	0.22	0.22
Health satisfaction	*	*	*	*	0.19	0.19
Finance security sat.	*	*	*	*	0.09	0.09
Future security sat.	*	*	*	*	0.15	0.15
Sense meaning sat.	*	*	*	*	0.14	0.14
Recreation sat.	*	*	*	*	0.17	0.17
Feel part comm sat.	*	*	*	*	0.07	0.07

* Not in equation, ** significance level too low to enter equation

respondents' health, financial security and sense of meaning in life most influential, each b = 0.16.

The first column of figures in Table 2.20 shows that 3 of 4 demographic variables remained statistically significant and collectively explained 4.0% of the variation in scores on the 5-item Satisfaction With Life Scale (SWLS). Of the three predictors, the most influential were household income and education, each b = 0.12. The second column of figures shows that only one of the 4 motivational indexes remained statistically significant and that explained 2.0% of the variance in SWLS scores. The Index of Arts as Community Builders (Comb) had a b = 0.14. The third column of figures shows that a single arts-related variable from the times per year set of predictors remained statistically significant, satisfaction obtained from going to non-art museums, b = 0.21, and it explained 4.0% of the variance in SWLS scores. The fourth column of figures shows that 6 of the domain satisfaction predictors remained statistically significant and together they explained 51.0% of the variance in SWLS scores. The most influential explanatory variables were satisfaction with respondents' sense of meaning in life and self-esteem, each b = 0.21, followed by satisfaction with respondents' health, b = 0.17. Again, the final column shows that the addition of each of the demographic and arts-related predictors to the 6 significant domain satisfaction predictors from the fourth column produced no change in our explanatory power. In our earlier study, we were able to explain 48.0% of the variance in SWLS scores, with satisfaction with one's financial security most influential, b = 0.22.

The first column of figures in Table 2.21 shows that two demographic variables remained statistically significant and explained 3.0% of the variation in scores on the 5-item Contentment with Life Assessment Scale (CLAS). Of the two predictors,

Table 2.20 Regressions of satisfaction with life scale (SWLS) on demographics, motivation indexes, hours/times engaged and satisfaction obtained from arts-related activities and domain satisfaction

Dependent variables	Demog.	Mot. Index	Times/sat.	Domain sat.	All Pred
N	487	582	308	534	534
% of variance expl	4	2	4	51	51
Predictors	b	b	b	b	b
Household income	0.12	*	*	*	**
Education	0.12	*	*	*	**
Age	0.11	*	*	*	**
Comm. Building Ind	*	0.14	*	*	**
Go other museums sat.	*	*	0.21	*	**
Sense meaning sat.	*	*	*	0.21	0.21
Job sat.	*	*	*	0.09	0.09
Health satisfaction	*	*	*	0.17	0.17
Finance security sat.	*	*	*	0.15	0.15
Feel part comm sat.	*	*	*	0.09	0.09
Self-esteem sat.	*	*	*	0.21	0.21

* Not in equation, ** significance level too low to enter equation

Table 2.21 Regressions of contentment with life assessment scale (CLAS) on demographics, motivation indexes, hours/times engaged and satisfaction obtained from arts-related activities and domain satisfaction

Dependent variables	Demog.	Times/sat.	Domain sat.	All Pred
N	493	353	538	538
% of variance expl	3	2	50	50
Predictors	b	b	b	b
Age	0.12	*	*	**
Household income	0.13	*	*	**
Singing alone sat.	*	*	*	**
Go historic site sat.	*	0.15	*	**
Job satisfaction	*	*	0.12	0.12
Health satisfaction	*	*	0.10	0.10
Self-esteem sat.	*	*	0.26	0.26
Future security sat.	*	*	0.18	0.18
Sense meaning sat.	*	*	0.16	0.16
Recreation act sat.	*	*	0.09	0.09

* Not in equation, ** significance level too low to enter equation

the most influential was household income, b = 0.13. The second column of figures shows that a single arts-related variable from the times per year set of predictors remained statistically significant, satisfaction obtained from visiting historic and heritage sites, b = 0.15, and explained 2.0% of the variance in CLAS scores. The third column of figures shows that 6 of the domain satisfaction variables remained statistically significant and together explained 50.0% of the variance in CLAS scores. The most influential explanatory variables were satisfaction with respondents' self-esteem, b = 0.26, followed by satisfaction with respondents' future security, b = 0.18. Again, the final column shows that the addition of each of the demographic and arts-related predictors to the 6 significant domain satisfaction predictors from the third column produced no change in our explanatory power. In our earlier study, we were able to explain 71.0% of the variance in CLAS scores, with satisfaction with respondents' financial security most influential, b = 0.19.

The first column of figures in Table 2.22 shows that two demographic variables remained statistically significant and explained 4.0% of the variation in scores on the 4-item Subjective Wellbeing Index (SWB). Of the two predictors, the most influential was household income, b = 0.17. The second column of figures shows that one of the 4 motivational indexes remained statistically significant and explained 2.0% of the variance in SWB scores. The Index of Arts as Community Builders had a b = 0.14. The third column of figures shows that a single arts-related variable from the hours per week set of predictors remained statistically significant, satisfaction obtained from reading novels, etc., b = 0.15, and explained 2.0% of the variance in SWB scores. The fourth column of figures shows that one arts-related variable from the times per year set of predictors remained statistically significant and explained 3.0% of the variance in SWB scores. Satisfaction obtained from going to art museums had a b = 0.17. The fifth column of figures shows that 9 of the domain satisfaction predictors remained statistically significant and together explained 75.0% of the variance in SWB scores. The most influential explanatory variables were satisfaction with respondents' financial security, b = 0.20, followed by satisfaction with

Table 2.22 Regressions of Subjective Wellbeing (SWB) on demographics, motivation indexes, hours/times engaged and satisfaction obtained from arts-related activities and domain satisfaction

Dependent variables	Demog.	Mot. Index	Hours/act.sat.	Times/sat.	Domain sat.	All Pred
N	491	583	423	374	644	644
% of variance expl	4	2	2	3	75	75
Predictors	b	b	b	b	b	b
Education	0.10	*	*	*	*	**
Household income	0.17	*	*	*	*	**
Comm. Building Ind.	*	0.14	*	*	*	**
Reading novels sat.	*	*	0.15	*	*	**
Go art museum sat.	*	*	*	0.17	*	**
Local treatment sat.	*	*	*	*	0.10	0.10
Friendships sat.	*	*	*	*	0.11	0.11
Future security sat.	*	*	*	*	0.13	0.13
Health satisfaction	*	*	*	*	0.19	0.19
Finance security sat.	*	*	*	*	0.20	0.20
Sense meaning sat	*	*	*	*	0.12	0.12
Self-esteem sat.	*	*	*	*	0.14	0.14
Recreation act sat.	*	*	*	*	0.12	0.12
Feel part comm sat.	*	*	*	*	0.06	0.06

* Not in equation, ** significance level too low to enter equation

respondents' health, b = 0.19. Again, the final column shows that the addition of each of the demographic and arts-related predictors to the 9 significant domain satisfaction predictors from the fifth column produced no change in our explanatory power. In our earlier study, we were able to explain 79.0% of the variance in SWB scores, with satisfaction with respondents' financial security most influential, b = 0.25.

Table 2.23 lists results of regressing our 7 life assessment variables on 7 mean respondent-calculated discrepancy scores. Although the predictors are drawn from multiple discrepancies theory (MDT), the whole theory is not applied here. All we have done is use the 7 basic discrepancy variables of MDT in a simple bottom-up type of linear regression of the sort applied to produce Exhibits 16–22. On average, the 7 MDT variables explained 44.0% (vs. 48.0% in the earlier study) of the variation in life assessment scores, with a high of 59.0% for SWLS and a low of 16.0% for GH. Without GH, the average variance explained was 49.0%. The difference between the power of the MDT variables to explain General Health versus the other 6 life assessment variables (replicating results in our earlier study) suggests again that respondents recognized a difference between a healthy life and a good life, all things considered. Setting aside the GH column, in every column, the most influential variable is that indicating the perceived discrepancy between what respondents have now and what they want. On average, the Beta value for this variable is b = 0.42, with a high of b = 0.46 for SWB and a low of b = 0.34 for qolsat. The only other MDT predictor with a significant association with each of the 7 life assessment variables in the presence of all other MDT predictors is that for the gap between what respondents have now and the best they ever had in the past. On average, this predictor had a b = 0.18.

Since in every case of Tables 2.16, 2.17, 2.18, 2.19, 2.20, 2.21, and 2.22, the set of domain satisfaction predictors explained the greatest amount of variance in our life assessment variables, the column headed 'Domain sat.' in these tables is the appropriate column to compare with the results in Table 2.23 in order to assess the relative explanatory power of both sets of predictors, i.e., domain satisfaction versus

Table 2.23 Regressions of seven life assessment variables on seven mean discrepancy scores

Dependent variables	GH	Lsat	hap	qolsat	SWLS	CLAS	SWB
N	657	656	657	656	641	636	645
% of variance explained	16	39	43	43	59	51	58
Predictors, your life compared to	b	b	b	b	b	b	b
What you want from life	0.17	0.42	0.43	0.34	0.43	0.41	0.46
What others your age & sex have	0.18	0.12	0.08	0.21	0.15	*	0.17
What you deserve	−0.12	*	*	*	0.08	0.09	0.09
What you need	*	*	*	0.11	0.10	0.08	0.09
What you expected it to be now	*	*	0.11	*	*	0.19	0.10
What you expect it to be in 5 years	*	*	*	*	*	*	*
The best in your past experience	0.23	0.22	0.18	0.15	0.20	0.13	0.13

* Significance level too low to enter equation

discrepancy predictors. On average for the 7 life assessment variables, domain satisfaction predictors clearly explained a greater percent of the variance than discrepancy predictors, 52.0 versus 44.0% (compared to 57 and 48% in the earlier study). This is not particularly surprising or satisfying since, after all, in the former case one is using only domain satisfaction predictors to explain some sort of a more general level of satisfaction. Much more analysis will be required to make a comprehensive comparison of the relative power of MDT versus a simple domain satisfaction, bottom-up approach to explaining the variation of overall life assessment scores in the context of a plausible theory that includes arts-related variables.

Conclusion

The aims of this investigation were (1) to measure the impact of arts-related activities on the perceived quality of life of a representative sample of British Columbians aged 18 years or more in the spring of 2007, and (2) to compare the findings of this study with those of a sample of 1027 adults drawn from 5 B.C. communities (Comox Valley, Kamloops, Nanaimo, Port Moody and Prince George) in the fall of 2006. In May and June 2007, 708 British Columbians responded to a 13-page mailed out questionnaire. The working data set was weighted by age and education to match the 2006 census statistics for the province, yielding a fairly representative sample.

Since we were aiming to get some baseline provincial figures as well as to replicate findings obtained from specifically targeted communities in different parts of the province, the best way to summarize our results is with a double column review. This is provided in Table 2.24. In broad strokes, out of 37 pairs of entries in this table, there are 10 (27.0%) in which the province-wide and five-communities results are the same. There are another 13 (35.0%) in which the results are very nearly the same. So, we have a total of 23 (62.0%) pairs with considerable similarity. While plenty of differences were identified in many of the tables in our main text, suggesting that there remains a great deal of diversity yet to be understood, the broad similarities seem to be quite remarkable.

In the light of results from our two samples and in the context of all our predictors, based on the relative impact of all the arts-related activities and the satisfaction obtained from those activities on the seven overall life assessment variables, it is fair to say that such activities and their corresponding satisfaction contributed relatively little. As remarked in our earlier study, it is important to keep in mind the initial condition, 'in the context of all our predictors' and the qualifier 'relatively'. In that context, even the usually powerful explanatory variables concerning interpersonal relations (i.e., satisfaction with one's living partner, family and friendships) had very little impact. Of the three, only satisfaction with one's friendships appeared in any final regression equation for the provincial sample and only for Lsat, Hap and SWB. This was quite different from the five-communities sample. In the latter, satisfaction with one's living partner appeared in the final equations for 6 of the 7 dependent variables (excluding General Health), satisfaction with family relations

Table 2.24 Comparisons between province-wide (2007, N = 708) and five-communities (2006, N = 1027) results

Province-wide sample	Five-communities sample
Top 5 arts-related hours per week activities: listening to music; reading novels, short stories, plays or poetry; watching films on DVD; singing alone; reading to others	Same
Top 5 arts-related hours per week activities: average hours per week engaged = 6.9	7.0
Top 5 arts-related hours per week activities: Average levels of satisfaction = 5.9	Same
Top 5 arts-related times per year activities: go to movies, concerts, community festivals, historic sites, art museums	Same
Top 5 arts-related times per year activities: average times per year going = 3.8	3.9
Top 5 arts-related times per year activities: average levels of satisfaction = 5.8	Same
First thoughts about 'arts' = painting, drawing	Same
Most important arts = music	Same
Place where first learned about arts = school	Same
Mean age when first learned = 12	12.7
Mean level of satisfaction with access to activity, information, place, access to place, price = 5.1	5.3
Mean level of satisfaction with support from city, provincial, federal government and others = 4.0	Same
Index of arts as self-health enhancers a = 0.87	0.88
Index of arts as self-developing activities a = 0.86	0.89
Index of arts as community builders a = 0.82	0.86
Index of arts as ends in themselves a = 0.71	0.77
Satisfaction with life scale (SWLS) a = 0.90	0.89
Contentment with life assessment scale (CLAS) a = 0.87	0.86
Subjective wellbeing index (SWB) a = 0.87	0.88
Average level of satisfaction on 30 domain/aspect items = 5.3	5.4
Average level of satisfaction with life as a whole, standard of living, quality of life and happiness = 5.8	Same
Top 2 discrepancy items = have/want, have/others have	Same

(continued)

Table 2.24 (continued)

Province-wide sample	Five-communities sample
Demographic variable with highest average correlation with 7 life assessment variables = household income, r = 0.12	r = 0.20
Hours per week arts-related variables with highest and second highest average correlations with 7 life assessment variables: satisfaction obtained from arranging flowers, r = 0.25; satisfaction obtained from taking kids to arts-related activities, r = −0.17	Satisfaction obtained from playing a musical instrument, r = 0.25; satisfaction obtained from singing in a group, r = 0.17
Life assessment variable with largest number of significant associations with hours per week arts-related variables: satisfaction with the overall quality of life tied with happiness	Satisfaction with the overall quality of life
Times per year arts-related variables with highest and second highest average correlations with 7 life assessment variables: satisfaction obtained from going to amateur theatre performances, r = 0.27; satisfaction obtained from going to professional theatre performances, r = 0.22	Satisfaction obtained from going to non-art museums, r = 0.14; satisfaction obtained from going to amateur theatre performances, r = 0.13
Life assessment variable with largest number of significant associations with times per year arts-related variables: Satisfaction with the overall quality of life	General health
Domain/aspect satisfaction items with highest and second highest average correlations with 7 life assessment variables: satisfaction with one's own health, r = 0.60; satisfaction with one's self-esteem, r = 0.59	Satisfaction with one's own health, r = 0.64; satisfaction with one's self-esteem, r = 0.57
Percent of variation explained in general health scores by all predictors = 20.0%, with most influential predictor = respondents' satisfaction with their recreation activities, b = 0.25	Percent of variation explained in general health scores by all predictors = 32.0%, with most influential predictor = respondents' satisfaction with their recreation activities, b = 0.28
Percent of variation explained in satisfaction with life as a whole scores (Lsat) by all predictors = 66.0%, with most influential predictor = respondents' satisfaction with their own health, b = 0.25	Percent of variation explained in satisfaction with life as a whole scores (Lsat) by all predictors = 71.0%, with most influential predictor = respondents' satisfaction with their own health, b = 0.24
Percent of variation explained in happiness scores by all predictors = 45.0%, with most influential predictor = respondents' satisfaction with their own self-esteem, b = 0.35	Percent of variation explained in happiness scores by all predictors = 51.0%, with most influential predictor = respondents' satisfaction with their Own health, b = 0.33

(continued)

Table 2.24 (continued)

Province-wide sample	Five-communities sample
Percent of variation explained in satisfaction with the overall quality of life scores (qolsat) by all predictors = 60.0%, with most influential predictor = respondents' satisfaction with their treatment by local residents, b = 0.22	Percent of variation explained in satisfaction with the overall quality of life scores (qolsat) by all predictors = 63.0%, with most influential predictors = respondents' satisfaction with their own health, financial security and sense of meaning in life, each b = 0.19
Percent of variation explained in satisfaction with life scale scores (SWLS) by all predictors = 51.0%, with most influential predictor = respondents' satisfaction with their own self-esteem and sense of meaning in life, b = 0.21	Percent of variation explained in satisfaction with life scale scores (SWLS) by all predictors = 48.0%, with most influential predictor = respondents' satisfaction with their financial security, b = 0.22
Percent of variation explained in contentment with life assessment scale scores (CLAS) by all predictors = 50.0%, with most influential predictor = respondents' satisfaction with their own self-esteem, b = 0.26	Percent of variation explained in contentment with life assessment scale scores (CLAS) by all predictors = 71.0%, with most influential predictor = respondents' satisfaction with their financial security, b = 0.19
Percent of variation explained in subjective wellbeing index scores (SWB) by all predictors = 75.0%, with most influential predictor = respondents' satisfaction with their financial security, b = 0.20	Percent of variation explained in subjective wellbeing index scores (SWB) by all predictors = 79.0%, with most influential predictor = respondents' satisfaction with their financial security, b = 0.25
Average percent of variation explained in 7 life assessment variables by all domain/aspect predictors = 52.0%	Average percent of variation explained in 7 life assessment variables by all domain/aspect predictors = 57.0%
Average percent of variation explained in 7 life assessment variables by 7 MDT predictors = 44.0%	Average percent of variation explained in 7 life assessment variables by 7 MDT predictors = 48.0%

appeared in the final equations for Lsat and Hap, and satisfaction with friendships appeared in the final equations for Lsat, qolsat and SWB.

Considering domain/aspect predictors, what did most of the explanatory work for the 7 life assessment variables? Two samples with 7 final regression equations and no ties would have given us 14 possible most influential predictors. Since we had one regression with a 3-way tie for most influential predictor and one with a 2-way tie, we have 17 entries. One way to answer our question is to count the relative frequency with which various predictors occur. Using this crude measure, one finds that satisfaction with financial security had 5 firsts, followed by 4 firsts for satisfaction with respondents' own health and 3 firsts for satisfaction with respondents' own self-esteem. These predictors are understandably and often relatively heavy hitters in such exercises. Still, granting the difficulties of displacing any of the relatively heavy hitters from our final explanatory equations, it remains unclear why even arts-related activities with engagement measured in the average number of hours per week or times per year and the satisfaction obtained from such engagement were relatively weak predictors in the context of only such arts-related activities and satisfaction. Hopefully, others will be able to solve this problem in the future.

Acknowledgments We would like to express our thanks to the Social Sciences and Humanities Research Council for funding this research through the Gold Medal for Achievement in Research 2004. This project complements an earlier one also funded by the Council through its Community-University Research grants program, with Will Garrett-Petts of Thompson Rivers University Principal Investigator. We would also like to thank Joyce Henley, Office Manager of ISRE, and all the anonymous respondents who shared their time and thoughts with us to make this report possible.

Appendix: BC Arts and Quality of Life Survey, May 2007

See Table 2.25

Table 2.25 Time spent on and levels of satisfaction with artistic activities (Total N = 708, unweighted data)

	Ordered by		
Particular activities	N	Hours/Week	Satisfaction
T1. Listening to music	608	13.22	6.01
T17. Reading novels, etc.	441	7.67	6.17
T37. Watching movies on video	278	4.96	5.60
T8. Singing alone	239	4.58	5.70
T21. Reading to others	195	3.27	6.03
T46. Gourmet cooking	136	4.60	6.18
T20. Telling stories	122	2.76	5.92
T5. Painting or drawing	118	5.86	5.97
T9. Singing in a group	103	2.67	6.11
T50. Watching art shows on TV	94	2.68	5.66
T2. Playing a musical instrument	85	4.91	6.05
T40. Artistic photography	66	3.11	6.34
T27. Knitting or crocheting	64	4.98	6.45
T42. Arranging flowers	57	1.37	6.38
T67. Other	50	10.00	6.65
T52. Watching concerts on TV	48	2.17	5.93
T12. Taking children to arts activities	46	2.35	5.96
T19. Writing novels, etc.	45	6.18	5.89
T28. Embroidery, needlepoint	38	5.95	6.31
T16. Making quilts	32	9.75	6.29

(continued)

Table 2.25 (continued)

Particular activities	Ordered by N	Hours/Week	Satisfaction
T15. Making clothes	30	4.27	6.07
T6. Teaching painting or drawing	23	5.13	6.05
T51. Watching live theatre on TV	23	2.48	5.42
T7. Teaching singing	21	3.90	6.05
T56. Attending a class-artistic work	20	3.65	6.39
T14. Designing clothes	17	2.47	5.94
T49. Graphic designing	17	16.29	5.63
T4. Teaching—to play an instrument	15	4.27	5.20
T24. Teaching people to dance	14	2.29	5.85
T43. Creating jewellery	14	2.64	5.56
T11. Creating sculptures	13	5.38	6.30
T47. Teaching gourmet cooking	13	2.85	6.30
T53. Watching opera on TV	12	3.17	5.38
T10. Creating pottery or ceramics	11	7.00	5.78
T18. Attending a book club	11	4.45	6.00
T60. Working for pay in the arts	10	26.80	6.22
T22. Teaching creative writing	9	2.33	5.63
T3. Writing music	7	4.43	5.57
T62. Acting as an advocate for the arts	7	1.71	6.33
T58. Selling works of art	6	2.33	5.83
T25. Weaving textiles	4	13.75	6.67
T35. Non-acting work—amateur theatre	2	2.50	6.50
T26. Weaving baskets	1	4.00	7.00
T34. Acting—amateur theatre	1	6.00	–
T48. Making artistic videos or movies	1	10.00	7.00
T61. Serving as a judge for the arts	1	2.00	–
T33. Acting—professional theatre	0		
T13. Teaching sculpture	0		
T36. Going to movies	439	5.97	5.53
T29. Going to concerts	417	3.75	6.01
T38. Going to art museums/galleries	384	3.65	5.84
T65. Visiting historic, heritage sites	367	2.97	5.93
T54. Attending community festivals	365	2.89	5.61
T39. Going to other museums	319	2.39	5.84
T66. Visiting the public library	307	9.18	5.61
T30. Going to amateur live theatre	296	2.56	5.90
T31. Going to professional live theatre	293	2.80	6.14
T57. Buying works of art	224	2.33	6.12
T44. Decorating a home	220	6.08	5.75
T32. Going to school plays	211	2.13	6.00
T23. Dancing	199	5.48	5.52
T41. Designing a garden	190	4.19	6.07

(continued)

Table 2.25 (continued)

	Ordered by		
Particular activities	N	Hours/Week	Satisfaction
T63. Making donations to the arts	111	2.62	5.79
T55. Working on community festivals	98	2.43	5.77
T59. Volunteering in the arts	53	4.94	5.94
T64. Designing, crafting furniture	49	4.16	6.02
T45. Figure skating	32	5.22	5.50
T67. Other	25	9.52	6.48
T61. Serving as a judge for the arts	8	3.00	6.14
T33. Acting—professional theatre	7	2.00	6.14
T34. Acting—amateur theatre	6	1.67	6.50
T60. Working for pay in the arts	10	26.80	6.22
T49. Graphic designing	17	16.29	5.63
T25. Weaving textiles	4	13.75	6.67
T1. Listening to music	608	13.22	6.01
T67. Other	50	10.00	6.65
T48. Making artistic videos or movies	1	10.00	7.00
T16. Making quilts	32	9.75	6.29
T17. Reading novels, etc.	441	7.67	6.17
T10. Creating pottery or ceramics	11	7.00	5.78
T19. Writing novels, etc.	45	6.18	5.89
T34. Acting—amateur theatre	1	6.00	–
T28. Embroidery, needlepoint	38	5.95	6.31
T5. Painting or drawing	118	5.86	5.97
T11. Creating sculptures	13	5.38	6.30
T6. Teaching painting or drawing	23	5.13	6.05
T27. Knitting or crocheting	64	4.98	6.45
T37. Watching movies on video	278	4.96	5.60
T2. Playing a musical instrument	85	4.91	6.05
T46. Gourmet cooking	136	4.60	6.18
T8. Singing alone	239	4.58	5.70
T18. Attending a book club	11	4.45	6.00
T3. Writing music	7	4.43	5.57
T4. Teaching—to play an instrument	15	4.27	5.20
T15. Making clothes	30	4.27	6.07
T26. Weaving baskets	1	4.00	7.00
T7. Teaching singing	21	3.90	6.05
T56. Attending a class-artistic work	20	3.65	6.39
T21. Reading to others	195	3.27	6.03
T53. Watching opera on TV	12	3.17	5.38
T40. Artistic photography	66	3.11	6.34
T47. Teaching gourmet cooking	13	2.85	6.30

(continued)

Table 2.25 (continued)

Particular activities	Ordered by		
	N	Hours/Week	Satisfaction
T20. Telling stories	122	2.76	5.92
T50. Watching art shows on TV	94	2.68	5.66
T9. Singing in a group	103	2.67	6.11
T43. Creating jewellery	14	2.64	5.56
T35. Non-acting work—amateur theatre	2	2.50	6.50
T51. Watching live theatre on TV	23	2.48	5.42
T14. Designing clothes	17	2.47	5.94
T12. Taking children to arts activities	46	2.35	5.96
T22. Teaching creative writing	9	2.33	5.63
T58. Selling works of art	6	2.33	5.83
T24. Teaching people to dance	14	2.29	5.85
T52. Watching concerts on TV	48	2.17	5.93
T61. Serving as a judge for the arts	1	2.00	–
T62. Acting as an advocate for the arts	7	1.71	6.33
T42. Arranging flowers	57	1.37	6.38
T33. Acting—professional theatre	0		
T13. Teaching sculpture	0		
T67. Other	25	9.52	6.48
T66. Visiting the public library	307	9.18	5.61
T44. Decorating a home	220	6.08	5.75
T36. Going to movies	439	5.97	5.53
T23. Dancing	199	5.48	5.52
T45. Figure skating	32	5.22	5.50
T59. Volunteering in the arts	53	4.94	5.94
T41. Designing a garden	190	4.19	6.07
T64. Designing, crafting furniture	49	4.16	6.02
T29. Going to concerts	417	3.75	6.01
T38. Going to art museums/galleries	384	3.65	5.84
T61. Serving as a judge for the arts	8	3.00	6.14
T65. Visiting historic, heritage sites	367	2.97	5.93
T54. Attending community festivals	365	2.89	5.61
T31. Going to professional live theatre	293	2.80	6.14
T63. Making donations to the arts	111	2.62	5.79
T30. Going to amateur live theatre	296	2.56	5.90
T55. Working on community festivals	98	2.43	5.77
T39. Going to other museums	319	2.39	5.84
T57. Buying works of art	224	2.33	6.12
T32. Going to school plays	211	2.13	6.00
T33. Acting—professional theatre	7	2.00	6.14
T34. Acting—amateur theatre	6	1.67	6.50

Most activities had some people indicating they spent a certain number of hours per week on it, while other people only did it a few times per year. The hours per week activities are listed first, followed by the times per year activities. The activities are listed in two orders—first from the largest number of people responding to the least and then from the largest average hours/week (or times/year) to the smallest.

References

Cummins, R. A., Stokes, M. A., & Davern, M. T. (2007). Core affect and subjective wellbeing: A rebuttal to Moum and Land. *Journal of Happiness Studies, 8*(4), 457–466. https://doi.org/10.1007/s10902-007-9065-2

Davern, M. T., Cummins, R. A., & Stokes, M. A. (2007). Subjective wellbeing as an affective-cognitive construct. *Journal of Happiness Studies, 8*(4), 429–449. https://doi.org/10.1007/s10902-007-9066-1

Decima. (2002). The arts in Canada: Access and availability, 2001 research study final report, Decima Research Inc., Ottawa. Accessed June 2007, from http://www.pch.gc.ca/progs/arts/pubs/etudereport/arts_access.pdf

Diener, E., Emmons, R. A., Larsen, R. J., & Griffin, S. (1985). The satisfaction with life scale. *Journal of Personality Assessment, 49*, 71–75. https://doi.org/10.1207/s15327752jpa4901_13

DiMaggio, P., & Pettitt, B. (1999). Surveys of public attitudes toward the arts: What surveys tell us about the arts' political trials—And how they might tell us even more. *Arts Education Policy Review, 100*(4), 32–37.

Land, K. C. (2007). Comments from Kenneth C. Land. *Journal of Happiness Studies, 8*(4), 455. https://doi.org/10.1007/s10902-007-9068-z

Lavallee, L. F., Hatch, P. M., Michalos, A. C., & McKinley, T. (2007). Development of the contentment with life assessment scale (CLAS): Using daily life experiences to verify levels of self-reported life satisfaction. *Social Indicators Research, 83*(2), 201–244. https://doi.org/10.1007/s11205-006-9054-6

Michalos, A. C. (1985). Multiple discrepancies theory (MDT). *Social Indicators Research, 16*(4), 347–413. https://doi.org/10.1007/BF00333288

Michalos, A. C. (1991). Global report on student Well-being. In *Life satisfaction and happiness* (Vol. 1). Springer-Verlag.

Michalos, A. C. (2004). Social indicators research and health-related quality of life research. *Social Indicators Research, 65*(1), 27–72. https://doi.org/10.1023/A:1025592219390

Michalos, A. C. (Ed.). (2005a). *Citation classics from social indicators research.* Springer Publishers.

Michalos, A. C. (2005b). Arts and the quality of life. *Social Indicators Research, 71*(1–3), 11–59. https://doi.org/10.1007/s11205-004-8013-3

Michalos, A. C., & Kahlke, P. M. (2008). Impact of arts-related activities on the perceived quality of life. *Social Indicators Research, 89*(2), 193–258. https://doi.org/10.1007/s11205-007-9236-x

Michalos, A. C., Thommasen, H. V., Read, R., Anderson, N., & Zumbo, B. D. (2005). Determinants of health and the quality of life in the Bella Coola Valley. *Social Indicators Research, 72*(1), 1–50. https://doi.org/10.1007/s11205-004-4512-5

Moum, T. (2007). A critique of 'subjective Wellbeing as an affective-cognitive construct. *Journal of Happiness Studies, 8*(4), 451–453. https://doi.org/10.1007/s10902-007-9067-0

Chapter 3
The Theatre as a Liminal Genre: Interferences Between a Social Indicator and a Social Agent

Arpad Szakolczai

Since at least the 1950s, research on social indicators is conducted in, and assumes, an empiricist-positivistic-quantitative epistemology, usually based on purposeful data collections.[1] However, it by no means should be so, and is even counterintuitive, as genuine social indicators simply *exist*; should be perceived, interpreted, and understood, and not 'produced' as 'facts' indeed (something that is made, *factum*); as they are rather genuine *data* (something as given, *datum*). The identification of research on social indicators with quantitative analysis is therefore a serious epistemological fallacy.[2]

This volume, however, is devoted to the theatre as a social indicator, and the theatre in fact, apart its other roles and functions, indeed can be interpreted as a special kind of social indicator in and of the modern world; almost a 'seismograph'.[3] Such special role is due to two reasons. To start with, the theatre not simply can be read as an 'indicator' of social life, but is a very particular, even extremely strong transformative agent of social life. The 'causality' of conventional social indicator

[1] It should be noted, however, that such perspective goes against the word and spirit of the work of Gabriel Tarde, a major though often ignored classic of sociology, who pioneered, from his own theoretical perspective, focusing on imitation—thus, having evident links with the theatre—research on 'social indicators'. See in particular Tarde (1969: 222–241).

[2] See Szakolczai (2023a) for details.

[3] On the thinker as a seismograph, see Aby Warburg (1999: 27). The idea of 'the architect as seismograph' was also central for Paolo Portoghesi (1931–2023), the great Italian architect who died recently. The close connection between the history of theatre and architecture goes back at least to the collaboration between Inigo jones and Ben Johnson (see Yates, 1975a).

A. Szakolczai (✉)
St Gallen Collegium, University of St Gallen, St. Gallen, Switzerland

University College Cork, Cork, Ireland
e-mail: a.szakolczai@ucc.ie

P. Corvo, I. Riccioni (eds.), *Theatre and Quality of Life*, Social Indicators Research Series 91, https://doi.org/10.1007/978-3-032-09731-6_3

research is strictly one-directional: the indicators supposedly inform us about the character of certain social processes, but do not interfere with them; do not alter social life. With theatre, the case is different: a particularly important theatrical performance certainly captured something fundamental in social life, this is why it encountered such a passionate response; but a theatrical presentation influences the state of mind, even moves the soul and spirit of the spectators, thus indirectly but in a possibly quite significant manner alters social life itself—when it does not directly provoke social change, or, as it was the case with Victor Hugo's *Hernani*, mentioning only one particularly relevant example, even spark a revolution. Thus, the theatre, just in the manner in which it is a powerful social indicator, is also a catalyst; or, in the terminology of Michel Serres (2014), between the theatre as revealing, in a quite unique manner, the 'state of soul' of a society, and the theatre as infecting society with mimetic desire, similarly to the infections of a parasite, there is a strange, mutual interplay or *interference*.

Furthermore, and beyond singling out for attention some milestone theatrical performances, the theatre was one of the most important though all but completely ignored factor in the rise of the modern world (Szakolczai, 2013). Mentioning here only one though particularly relevant example, the 'public sphere', championed by Habermas with particular zeal is not simply the area for rational discussion, but is a fundamentally theatrical arena, which people enter in masks in order to play strategic games. The rise of the modern public sphere and of the theatre was deeply intertwined, back to their joint late Renaissance fairground origins, incorporating in a central way the rise of the modern economy, technology, and science as well.

The history, and the present, of the theatre therefore indeed offers a genuine goldmine of information about social processes and the state of the social world. However, here it should be immediately noted that theatricalised forms of conduct, and in particular the promotion of theatricalisation, as the reference to the 'public sphere' already indicated, encompass areas way beyond the theatre. Here an entire line of development can be indicated, in a sketch: in a series of evermore accelerating changes in the twentieth century, the theatre yielded its place to the cinema, which by the 1980s itself was overtaken by video-recorders, a practice that, after a victorious march lasting a couple of decades was itself replaced by the Internet—and basically this is where we now are, at a particular end-station, or rather 'endgame' (Beckett).

Given the focus of this book on the theatre, and not its heirs, and given the tight word limits, the paper will focus on three instances of theatre as social indicator and catalyst: Shakespeare, Molière and Bulgakov.

First, however, a few comments will be offered on the liminal character of the theatre, which much helps to understand its role as both a social indicator and a catalyst.

The Theatre as a Liminal Genre

It is not a new idea to claim that the theatre is a liminal place, and so genre. It was formulated paradigmatically by Victor Turner, a main theorist of liminality, even evoked in the title of one of his books, *From Ritual to Theatre*.

The liminal character of the theatre can be seen by starting from the classic definition of Peter Brook, but read it through Agnes Horvath's (2021) ingenious interpretation of liminality. According to Brook, for a theatrical performance nothing else is needed than an empty space in which some people appear while others watch them. We only need to add, through Agnes Horvath, that such an empty space is nothing else than a liminal void; or a void which for some reason is pregnant with meaning, past or present; where something is bound to happen. Such focus on the void definitely moves away from Victor Turner's 'liminoid' interpretation of the theatre, and closer to the original perspective of van Gennep (1960), according to whom the archetypal rite of passage and thus liminal moment was not an initiation rite of adolescents, rather burial, thus again a kind of void experience.

The specific void character of the theatre becomes visible if we explore the close analogies between theatre and painting. A painting is two-dimensional, while a theatrical performance is three-dimensional, so this would suggest to search for parallels with three-dimensional sculpture, but this is misleading, as a sculpture can be beheld from every side, while the spectator is fixed in a seat in a theatrical performance, just as the beholder of an image must focus his attention in a specific, fixed manner on a pre-set space of the image. This, in fact, is the second main parallel between theatre and painting: just as theatre, painting also starts with an empty space, the delimination of a void square, onto which the painter conjures up the image.

One might say that this takes for granted modern oil painting, but this is not the case. The point is not simply that in this regard Chinese or Japanese art proceeds in a more or less identical manner, but that the very first painted images, on cave walls, also have a close connection to the void: a cave is nothing else but a void, a kind of womb inside the Earth, and the cave paintings were placed on the walls containing this void, having an eerie parallel both with theatre and later, formal painting. The affinity with theatre was indeed explored already in the Palaeolithic, as evidently some kind of ritualistic-theatrical performances, using music, were performed in the painted caves (Montelle, 2009).

The theatre, thus, is not just a liminal space, and is also more than a modern, liminoid version of the 'classical' liminal rituals (Turner, 1982): it is a full-scale liminal phenomenon, or—using the terminology of Goethe, a great theatre person, among others—has a particular 'elective affinity' with liminality. This means that the theatre is a particularly sensitive social indicator, or is a genuine 'seismograph' of coming liminal situations; however, at the same time, when signalling liminality, it can itself anticipate or even provoke liminal situations, can thus be a magnifier or agent of liminality, and at its most dangerous level it can contribute to the theatricalisation of social life, or can help to turn liminality, through abusing the elective affinity, into a permanent condition.[4]

A perfect example for the affinity between theatre and liminality is offered by the most famous playwright of all times, William Shakespeare.

The Liminal Theatre of Shakespeare: Magic and Infectious Desire

It is well known that Shakespeare lived on the threshold of a major period of transition, or liminal moment, of European history, between the Renaissance and the early modern period, himself being torn between Catholic and Protestant allegiances in his family. However, both the nature of this liminal moment and the significance of Shakespeare can be rendered more precise through a formulation of Frances Yates: 'History falls inexorably into "periods": for Europe as a whole it divides into the Renaissance and the seventeenth century; for England, it divides into the Elizabethan age and the Stuart age. In this periodisation, the important interstices tend to be overlooked, the times between the periods, times when survivors of an earlier period are still alive and influential, times when an earlier period has not fully ceased and the new period is not yet fully born. The first fifteen or so years of the seventeenth century were such a time in all Europe' (1975a: 80). Yates was a historian of science and of the related rationalistic method, but the same period also turned out to be vital for the rise of modern politics and economics, identified as central by Michel Foucault (1981), concerning the rise of the police and the idea of the reason of state, and through Foucault it can be extended, following Joyce Appleby (1978), to economic thinking.[5] The main works of Shakespeare are exact contemporaries of these developments.

If we take Shakespeare's theatre as a 'social indicator', or as revealing the inner state (*stato d'anima*) of a particular community, then it first of all shows a world completely at the mercy of contagious imitative or mimetic processes. This is the central theme of the Shakespeare book of the great contemporary theorist of imitation, René Girard (2004). Imitativity pervades every level of social life, as staged by Shakespeare, from the micro sphere of intimate relations, especially love, up to the macro level of societal relations, and even the conflicts between states, or international relations: everything is guided by mimetic desires and imitative rivalries, which are spinning each other, both upwards and downwards, inside social life, and

[4] This point is taken up in Szakolczai (2023b).

[5] The first four treatises on something like 'economics', some even baptising it as 'political economy', an expression which for Aristotle was deprived of any sense, were written in France in between 1599 and 1615 by Huguenots: Barthélemy de Laffemas, Olivier de Serres, Louis Turquet de Mayerne, and Antoine de Montchrétien; Schumpeter (1954) mistakenly prioritises Montchrétien, the only one he mentions. The English writers discussed by Appleby (1978) started to write in the 1620s, but 'after the fact'. For further details, see Szakolczai (2023a, Ch5).

which are even infesting supposedly rational conducts, as the transformation of every social relation into parts in purposeful strategic games, advancing contemporary game theory, is just the reverse side of mimetic rivalries, have nothing to do with genuine reason and understanding. This is particularly visible in one of Shakespeare's most extraordinary and least understood plays, *Troilus and Cressida*, where, as an important and innovative reading of the Trojan War, sparked anyway by seduction of Helen, a woman who combined extraordinary 'beauty with easy infidelity',[6] the play is continuously shifting between the different levels of mimetic desires and strategic rivalries. Here Shakespeare is offering a truly Platonic reading of Homer, turning the *Iliad* from a presumed celebration of the heroism of warfare into an ironic tale, occasionally even outright a farce; a play which arguably was not properly understood until the First World War, and by the soldiers returning from the front.[7]

Contagious imitativity requires agents who spark or spin such processes, and this is done by the protagonist of the play for Girard, especially as seen from our contemporary eyes: Pandarus, a genuine trickster figure. Pandarus is a go-between who brings together Troilus and Cressida, literally procuring the bed where they unite. He stands for eliciting desire, kindling it where it does not exist, and then whip it up continuously, in ever increasing spirals, until his victims lose all control of themselves. In this quality, Pandaros becomes 'the midwife and engineer of desire' (Girard, 2004: 123). Moving way beyond a simple pimp, he 'takes a giant step forward' and, like Renaissance charlatans, '[i]nstead of waiting for his customers to show up, he generates them through advertising, creat[ing] his own markets' (152). The language used is not accidental, as Girard considers Pandarus 'a prophet of modern advertising', who recognised the effectiveness of spin control or 'sexiness by proxy' (123). Lines in the play recall modern-day media advisors addressing politicians, or even 'the way popular hosts handle their guests on TV shows' (148); an observation which leads Girard to introduce terms like 'pandaric methods' (149), or the 'pandarisation' of social life: 'At the end of the play everybody is turning into a Pandarus, everybody is trying to use for its own advantage the contagious forces that rule the world of warfare, politics and sex through the same mimetic strategies' (157). Girard singles out for attention one aspect of the 'Pandaric method', the technique of repetition: 'Constant harping on the same theme will trigger imitation more or less automatically' (125); the same method identified in the literature on tricksters.[8] In sum, '[i]f the industry needs a patron saint, it should select Pandarus' (123). Pandarus helps Girard making the point that he is not imposing his own theory of mimetic desire on Shakespeare, but Shakespeare himself was a theoretician of mimetic desire (121).

---

[6] '*la facilità al tradimento e la bellezza*'; Calasso (1988: 155).

[7] See Hyland (1989). See also the transliteration of Homer by Robert Graves (*The Anger of Achilles: The Iliad*), who himself was such a soldier, in WWI.

[8] For details, see Horvath (2013).

In a world infected by contagious imitation people feel sick, mentally and spiritually, and such sickness is indeed diagnosed by Shakespeare, as melancholy. Melancholy is not simply an individual condition, but sign of deeper social, even civilisational pathologies; and while it is clearly a troublesome condition, it is also a paradoxical anti-illness, as a melancholic person is not simply 'sick', but literally and technically a 'non-sick sick'. Melancholy challenges the limits between illness and health, body and spirit, individual and social order. It is to feel sad or gloomy without a reason; it is to consider life itself as a burden. Melancholy is a psychological condition, yet it has evident social correlates, as it is contagious: for centuries it hardly appears, and then suddenly spreads as an epidemic. Here again Shakespeare was a particularly perceptive seismograph, as Robert Burton's classic *The Anatomy of Melancholy* appeared in 1621. Melancholy proliferates in moments of transition; it is a disease of transitions, including transitions to modernity, especially the transitionality of modernity as a movement towards permanent liminality.[9] Several protagonists of *The Merchant of Venice* suffer from melancholy, as if that was a contagious disease, but the most melancholy character of all is Jaques, from *As You Like It*. They are indeed key, representative figures of Shakespeare's life-work as a seismograph, so must be discussed in some further detail.[10]

The figures are literally 'representative', as they are taken from the two main fields that serve as if incubators of modern permanent liminality, thus showing a particularly strong dose of melancholy, economy and the theatre. *The Merchant of Venice*, most evidently, is about merchants, or the main agents of the exchange economy, that was just emerging in Shakespeare's time as not simply a specific and rather marginal field of social life, but its new centre, starting to spin everything else—even identifying Venice as the place through which, from the Byzantium, mercantile-commercial mentality spread throughout Europe.[11] Commerce is about the exchange of some objects to others, through the intermediary of money, thus is an instrument of substitution. This could only be extended to an ever larger area of social life if people are induced to an ever larger area of their life, activities and possession as substitutable thus interchangeable, which implies the spread of imitativity, undermining meaning, while also implying risks, spinning further uncertainty, liminality and melancholy. The eponymous protagonists of the play, the *real* merchants of Venice, just as 'the' merchant of Venice, Shylock, are spinning such substitutive imitativity in their different ways, entrapped in a trickster logic, the same as being spun by Pandarus, paying the price of melancholy and/or hardened heart, while also forgetting the natural *charis* logic of social life. This is reasserted in the

[9] The connections between melancholy and modernity were studied by two important contemporary social theorists, Wolf Lepenies (1992) and Harvie Ferguson (1995). For further discussion, see Szakolczai (2017, Ch7).

[10] Interestingly, *As You Like It* was the first main success of the Kaposvár Theatre, with which they competed in the Theatre of Nations festival in Warsaw in 1975 (see Szakolczai, 2023b).

[11] The next key stage in this regard in the history of the theatre was 'domestic tragedy', highlighted by Edward Moore and George Lillo, in the early eighteenth century, promoting the social acceptance of merchants. For details, see Szakolczai (2015).

great monologue of Portia, the culmination of the play, also delivering the judgment on the trickster logic by which all merchants live, as it conclusively asserts that human flesh, or the real, concrete substance of human beings cannot be quantified exactly, and so such quantification, central for exchange and substitutability, has no sense whatsoever for human life.

Through Jaques, indirectly, but in a most important manner, Shakespeare identifies the second main agent of infectious imitativity, the theatre.[12] Here Girard must be complemented by the similarly milestone work of Ted Hughes (1992). Hughes ingenuously argues that Jaques is not simply an evidently autobiographical character, but this is even revealed by his name, as Jaques is the French version of James, which through its Catholic-Irish modality as Seamus, thus as Jaques-Seamus, plays with Shakespeare's own name. The conjecture gains its full weight by realising that Iago is the Spanish version of James, so it belongs to the same equation—except that Iago is one of the worst villains in Shakespeare, so it becomes quite paradoxical to argue for *its* own autobiographical character. This, however, can be done by realising that a subtle change in modality happens in the movement from Jaques to Iago: Jaques presents Shakespeare as the victim of unleashed imitative processes, while with Iago Shakespeare moves from victim to perpetrator. The solution is that in this way Shakespeare identifies the theatre as a main agent of imitativity: the contagious imitativity that captured Shakespeare when young, making him prone to melancholy; while once he became a playwright, especially the writer of comedies, he himself became the agent of spreading such contagious processes, both mimetic desire but also uncontrollable jealousy, inside society. The highly autobiographical plays around 1600 made him fully aware of the problems involved in his own activities, and as a result he stopped staging comedies, instead writing and producing the four most important tragedies in world theatre, exploring what happens in the world when desire and ambition turn limitless, just when hypocrisy becomes all-pervasive, and so all stable reference points vanish into thin air.

Shakespeare's diagnosis of his own times, and the responsibility of the theatre, reaches its culmination in his very last play, *The Tempest*. The play is about a *par excellence* liminal situation, the storm and its aftermath; it also takes place in a *par excellence* liminal location, an island. Its hero, Prospero, widely recognised as one of the most autobiographical figures of Shakespeare, is a magician, and in him Frances Yates (1975) outright recognises the most important English Renaissance scientist-mathematician magician, John Dee, a paradoxical 'archetypal' figure of Bacon, Descartes and Newton. Prospero uses his magic to entrap Antonio, his brother who did him wrong, thus for a no doubt 'rightful' reason. Everything goes according to his plan, his enemies are immobilised and delivered to his mercy—but exactly at this point something clicks in his mind, and he not only fails to exact revenge but, once he managed to arrange matters for the best, gives up his magic altogether, dismantling his servants and instruments. The significance of this act is

[12] On the tight connection between the economy and theatre as agents of social transformation, see Agnew (1986).

visible through the way he imitated in his real life what Shakespeare announced in the theatre: he, Shakespeare now and not Prospero, also dismissed his own magic forever, and stopped writing and acting theatrical plays.

The corollary is crystal clear, and as if advances the anthropology of Alfred Gell: theatre, just as technologized-mathematical science, based on the operations of the zero, is a form of magic, and an infective one; it works very well, manages to infect and transform people, but exactly for this reason it is an extremely dangerous play, and should be simply abandoned. Shakespeare thus has an extremely important message for us: it is not simply that we must stop playing theatre, but that we moderns must stop fooling around with technologised art and science and its magical but ultimately self-destructive as infective tricks. Thus, Shakespeare is indeed our contemporary (Kott, 1964)[13]—and in its last part, the paper will offer some suggestions why this was prominently recognised by an East-European interpreter.

The Liminal Theatre of Molière: The Infectious Hypocrisy of an Exchange Society

The next great playwright after Shakespeare, in chronological as well as absolute order, was Molière (1622–1673). Molière lived through the next great liminal moment of European history, the rise of the absolute states after the liminal void generated by Thirty Years War, and in particular acting as the court comedian of the greatest absolute ruler, Louis XIV the Sun King (1638–1715), in the starting decades of his adult rule. His plays therefore jointly addressed the two great socio-political developments rooted in the liminal decades around 1600, the rise of the exchange economy and the absolute state driven by reason of state and building up its police. Here I'll use as guide Michel Serres, another key French contemporary thinker, first close colleague of Michel Foucault, and then a life-long friend of René Girard.

If, following Girard, Shakespeare was primarily a diagnost of modern infectious mimetic desire, then, following Serres, Molière was primarily a diagnost of a parallel development, endemic hypocrisy, and so even outright a theorist of modernity. Thus, a key essay with the stunning title 'Apparition of Hermes: Dom Juan', concluding chapter to *Hermes I*, his first book after his thesis, and introductory chapter to the first English collection of his writings (Serres, 1982), makes it evident that Molière's hero is a trickster figure: communication—which is not identical to language, according to key, foundational linguistic anthropologists like Edward Sapir and Benjamin Lee Whorf—is the primary realm of the trickster. Dom Juan is also characterised as a 'first hero of modernity', being at once a man of desire, a man of discourse and a man of money, but also a 'scientific observer of society', or a

[13] For a crucial modern reading of *The Tempest*, see W.H. Auden, 'The Sea and the Mirror: A commentary on Shakespeare's *The Tempest*', written in the middle of WWII. It is also centrally devoted to the disillusioned illusionist, one of his key lines being 'Ariel, I am that I am, your late and lonely master,/ Who knows now what magic is:—the power to enchant/ That comes from disillusion'.

sociologist *avant la lettre*—a title which evidently falls back to Molière. This is justified by Molière's analysis of the modern world in the making, captured as a society obsessed with exchange and substitution, thus a bunch of primitives, applying Mauss' idea of primitive gift exchange. This, however, cannot be accepted as a correct reading of Mauss, as the term 'gift exchange' is an unfortunate lapse in Mauss: gifts cannot be exchanged, only given, at most 'circulated' in a sense, and Mauss made such gift giving and not 'gift exchange' foundational for his kind of sociology. The modern obsession with exchange and substitution can rather be termed, through Michel Henry (2001), as an evidence of re-barbarisation, a fall from an acquired level of culture or civilisation.

Such obsession has evident theatrical affinities, through the close links between exchange, substitution and theatricality: the spectators in a theatre closely recall the customers of a fair, who first of all also indeed assist to all kinds of fairground spectacles, origins of modern theatre just as modern advertisement and the media in general, while the exchange of goods in fairs and markets assume the same kind of substitutability as between the roles played by actors on stage and by the 'actors' of an exchange society. So what Molière set on stage is this kind of society itself, with the actors, or the puppets reflecting the spectators; in other words, the spectators are themselves the puppets on the stage. The corollary is that a society where human life and social life are rendered substitutable through the ubiquity of exchange, helped by the theatre, is also a society of hypocrites.

A society of hypocrites is produced by exchange and theatricality in a series of steps. The first is the transformation of the community into spectators, isolated in the dark and closed into themselves, in a manner strikingly recalling Foucault and the Panopticon.[14] Second, in such a quasi-alchemic incubator, metamorphosis runs amok and the spectators establish all kind of identity-substitution games with stage characters—identifying with them, thus substituting themselves; or by turning the characters impersonated, even the actors/actresses themselves into objects of desire through fantasies of wish-fulfilment. In the third stage, the concrete social dynamics of lived life and gift-relations gradually yield their place, through depersonalisation and decontextualisation, to the kind of behaviour characteristic of exchange societies: rational strategic games to pursue the incited aims of mimetic desires. This has fundamental corollaries both for reason and ethic: in an exchange-substitution society reason becomes reduced to the pursuit of strategic games, trying to defeat the other, instead of building sociability through natural benevolence in pursuit of the good life of Plato and Aristotle; while moral principles become merely hypocritical façades, in an existentially corrupt society pervaded by self-designated 'do-gooders' (*buonismo*). The ultimate play presenting on stage the main characters of such a hypocritical society was *Tartuffe*, which showed how the clergy itself came to play a role in this society of hypocrites, and which became the ultimate play about the parasitic character of such a society, drawing predictable, furious hostility.

[14] Such affinities were recognised in some histories of the theatre. The incubator-like character of cinema was identified by Thomas Mann in his *Magic Mountain*.

The ultimate step of such a diagnosis, moving towards hyper-modernity and its permanent liminality, is offered in *Dom Juan*, by the contrasting characterisation of the hero by Sganarelle and the protagonist himself. Sganarelle, one of Molière's central characters, always played by himself,[15] offers the classical unmasking of the hero as a fake and hypocrite. Dom Juan, however, characterising himself, moves much further: he does not simply fake to follow the main values of culture, like beauty, love or nature, but one by one empties them of meaning, by pursuing them through brutal, objectifying conquest and destructive metamorphosis. In his other essays, Serres pursues this point, leading to science and technology, though not through Molière, as—in contrast to Shakespeare—it is not there in his plays, but among others through Bacon and Descartes, demonstrating the thorough theatricality of modern rationalism.

Molière's presentation of the world of absolutist France under Louis XIV as a society of hypocrites, also explored for sociological analysis by Norbert Elias as the ideal-type of a 'court society', was taken up in another key 'chronotope' (Bakhtin) of modernity, Stalinist Bolshevism in the 1920s and 1930s.

The Liminal Theatre of Bulgakov: Cabals and Hypocrites

Turning to classics in order to tell what otherwise could not be told was a main trope in the world beyond the Iron Curtain, and Bulgakov used Molière for such purposes several ways. Most important of these was the play *The Cabal of Hypocrites* (Bulgakov 2017), culmination and also end of his theatrical career, as the play was taken off after seven sold-out performances, and Bulgakov was never allowed to stage another play.

Both title words are of exceptional significance, even though this original title had to be abandoned so that the play, after a delay of several years, could finally be staged. The word 'hypocrite' speaks for itself, central term for the historical Molière, and also for the way Bulgakov attempted to make him actual to his time and place, also evident in his biography of Molière (Bulgakov, 1969), where the staging of Tartuffe plays a major role. The word 'cabal', however, is not there in Molière, it is Bulgakov's own revealing, piercing insight into his own world, with lasting significance for ours.

In the play, the 'cabal' is organised by a group of churchmen, making appearance only in the Third Act—in the opening Act Molière appears as Sganarelle, with both Pulcinella and a charlatan making appearance—both figures being historically central in launching modern trickster logic through the fairground and theatre. However, neither the Western nor the Eastern churches operated as cabals, with the possible exception of the Inquisition, but this was irrelevant for the times of Louis XIV, while

[15] Etymology, as always, is revealing: the name can be traced to Italian *sgannare*, or to 'disillusion' by unmasking—most paradoxically, by a theatrical mask.

plotting churchmen were completely so for Stalinist Russia. This was clearly not Bulgakov's interest: the churchmen were only thinly disguised masks for the ideologues of the Bolshevik regime.

But still, why a cabal? After all, in Bolshevik Russia Communist ideologues did not need to conspire in the background; they were themselves in power. And yet, the allusion evidently worked; they felt themselves hit. This was partly because of ingrained habit—Communist ideologues had to conspire in the past. However, the main point and the reason of the hit was not historical, rather that they *still* kept behaving in the same way, even when in power; and this mode of behaving applied particularly well to Bulgakov's main enemies, as also presented in the contemporary *Theatrical Novel*, published in English as *Black Snow*: the critics. In other words, and amazingly, the main place for cabals was the media, or the supposedly wide and open public sphere.[16] And this insight has vital relevance even for our present days, having a close affinity with Koselleck's *Critique and Crisis*, and also Heimito von Doderer's *Demons*, a work which has a Russian inspiration, as it was modelled on Dostoevsky's *Demons*: the modern 'political' organisations that function most closely on the principle of a cabal, back to their coffee house days, and shared with their close bedfellow, the stock-market, are the various medias.

Conclusion

Being a liminal genre, theatre is a particularly good indicator of liminal moments or processes in social life. However, due to the same, it is also a potentially quite problematic source of liminal transformations, as modes of behaviour set on stage can provoke lasting changes inside social life, turning theatre, and its technologised heirs, in a nick of time, from a social 'indicator' to an agent of infection. In all these, the theatre has a particularly close affinity with the medias.

In so far as the media mostly meant printed journals, theatricalisation and mediatisation were relatively independent processes. However, the more both theatres and printed media were complemented, and increasingly all but replaced, by their thoroughly mechanised, depersonalised and technologised versions, the more the two became conflated, and in a most dangerous and unhealthy manner, as the informative, even revelatory, and the infective-transformatory aspects became ever more mixed, promoting ever further a theatricalisation of social life—almost without any genuine theatre. A revisitation of some of the main chronotopes in the history of the theatre hopefully can help us to understand the important but also highly ambivalent role of the theatre, and close genres, in both diagnosing and promoting the

[16] On the media as a void place of parasites, see Niebisch (2012); see also Frances Yates' (1975b) focus on the Rosicrucians as the first case for the use and abuse of the rising public sphere. Yates underlines their significance by her title, invoking the Enlightenment, and also by associating both Bacon and Descartes with the Rosicrucians. Descartes was also associated with the Rosicrucians by Aldous Huxley (1982: 240).

theatricalisation of social life—or the emergence of a hypocritical society, infected by parasites and driven by a trickster logic, instead of the natural sociability of a *charis* logic, characteristic of archaic-primitive societies—constituting the most recent of the many historical lapses into barbarism.

References

Agnew, J.-C. (1986). *Worlds apart: The market and the theater in Anglo-American thought, 1550-1750*. Cambridge University Press.

Appleby, J. (1978). *Economic thought and ideology in seventeenth-century England*. Princeton University Press.

Bulgakov, M. (1969). *Vita del signor di Molière*. Mondadori.

Bulgakov, M. (2017). *Molière, or the cabal of hypocrites and Don Quixote: Two plays*. Theatre Communications Group.

Calasso, R. (1988). *Le nozze di Cadmo e Armonia*. Adelphi.

Ferguson, H. (1995). *Melancholy and the critique of modernity: Soren Kierkegaard's religious psychology*. Routledge.

Foucault, M. (1981). Omnes et Singulatim: Towards a criticism of "political reason". In S. M. McMurrin (Ed.), *The Tanner lectures on human values*. The University of Utah Press.

Girard, R. (2004). *The theatre of envy*. St Augustine's Press.

Henry, M. (2001). *La barbarie*. PUF.

Horvath, A. (2013). *Modernism and charisma*. Palgrave.

Horvath, A. (2021). *Political alchemy: Technology unbounded*. Routledge.

Hughes, T. (1992). *Shakespeare and the goddess of complete being*. Faber.

Huxley, A. (1982). *Grey Eminence: A study in religion and politics*. Triad/Granada. [1944].

Hyland, P. (1989). *Shakespeare: Troilus and Cressida*. Penguin.

Kott, J. (1964). *Shakespeare our contemporary*. Norton.

Lepenies, W. (1992). *Melancholy and society*. Harvard University Press.

Montelle, Y.-P. (2009). *Paleoperformance: The emergence of theatricality as social practice*. Seagull.

Niebisch, A. (2012). *Media parasites in the early Avant-Garde: On the abuse of technology and communication*. Palgrave.

Schumpeter, J. A. (1954). *History of economic analysis*. Oxford University Press.

Serres, M. (1982). *Hermes: Science, literature, philosophy*. John Hopkins University Press.

Serres, M. (2014). *Le parasite*. Fayard. [1980].

Szakolczai, A. (2013). *Comedy and the public sphere: The re-birth of theatre as comedy and the genealogy of the modern public arena*. Routledge.

Szakolczai, A. (2015). The Theatricalisation of the social: Problematising the public sphere. *Cultural Sociology, 9*(2), 220–239.

Szakolczai, A. (2017). *Permanent liminality and modernity: Analysing the sacrificial carnival through novels*. Routledge.

Szakolczai, A. (2023a). *Political anthropology as method*. Routledge.

Szakolczai, A. (2023b). Coping with permanent liminality: Social understanding and action through theatre in late communist Hungary. *Social Sciences, 12*(12), 652.

Tarde, G. (1969). *On communication and social influence*. (Terry N. Clark, Ed.). The University of Chicago Press.

Turner, V. (1982). *From ritual to theatre: The human seriousness of play*. PAJ Publications.

Van Gennep, A. (1960). *The rites of passage*. Chicago University Press. [1909].

Warburg, A. (1999). *The renewal of pagan antiquity*. Getty Research Institute.
Yates, F. (1975a). *Shakespeare's last plays*. Routledge.
Yates, F. (1975b). *The Rosicrucian enlightenment*. Paladine Books. [1972].

Chapter 4
Social Implications in Amleto

Paolo Corvo

Introduction

Approaching *Hamlet* from a sociological perspective may appear audacious, since the analysis of a literary text requires specific competences. Nevertheless, Shakespeare's tragedy lends itself to such an approach because it is rich in political and social references. As this essay will show, *Hamlet* is perhaps Shakespeare's most "sociological" work, addressing themes such as identity, reflexivity, and the relationship between the individual, justice, and power.

Hamlet, Prince of Denmark, is not merely the protagonist of a revenge tragedy, but a cultural icon that, although born in the Renaissance, continues to question us about the nature of modern subjectivity. Shakespeare's play does not merely narrate a story of intrigue and murder; it constitutes a profound meditation on the crisis of identity, on the irreconcilable conflict between thought and action, and on the crushing weight of conscience in a world that has lost its certainties. In this sense, Hamlet is the forerunner of modern man: an individual who can no longer rely on an ordered universe or a predetermined destiny, but is forced to define himself in a void of values and within a reality permeated by dissimulation. His tragedy is the tragedy of a keen mind which, instead of acting, consumes itself in reflection, in the search for a truth that seems unattainable (Bertinetti, 2021).

If the Renaissance still had faith in reason as a tool to order the world, Hamlet inaugurates the season of uncertainty: the mind as a space of conflict rather than synthesis. This tension is fully recognisable today in the experience of individuals who, immersed in globalised, hyper-connected, and plural societies, are compelled to define themselves continually in the face of shifting scenarios and contradictory norms (Giddens, 1991).

P. Corvo (✉)
University of Gastronomic Sciences, Bra-Pollenzo, CN, Italy
e-mail: p.corvo@unisg.it

P. Corvo, I. Riccioni (eds.), *Theatre and Quality of Life*, Social Indicators Research Series 91, https://doi.org/10.1007/978-3-032-09731-6_4

This essay aims to explore Hamlet's modernity through a primarily sociological lens, analysing the character as the embodiment of a subject alienated, fragmented, and oppressed by the complexity of social expectations. His figure is not that of a hero fighting external forces, but of an individual struggling against his own being, against uncertainty, and against the obligation to act in a context devoid of meaning. His inaction is not a sign of weakness, but the representation of an existential paralysis that resonates deeply with contemporary experience.

The Court of Elsinore: A Sociology of Power and Social Control

The famous line *"Something is rotten in the state of Denmark"* is not a mere metaphor. It is the diagnosis of an entire social and political structure in decay, a diseased system whose roots lie in a crime that is both political and familial. The assassination of the old King Hamlet is an act that cannot be easily repaired, and the new king, Claudius, knows this well. For this reason, he does not rely on brute force or overt repression, but on a sophisticated manipulation of consensus and control.

He does not establish an obvious regime of terror, but builds his authority through cultural manipulation and the concealment of truth.

Claudius's power is, in this sense, eminently modern: it rests on appearance, rhetoric, and the management of information. The court is an architecture of surveillance and dissimulation, a place where lies are the most common currency and the real crime is to refuse to conform to the fiction of power.

This form of power, which acts at the symbolic level, was analysed by Pierre Bourdieu (2001) as *symbolic violence*, that is, the ability to impose a vision of the world and to have one's authority accepted as legitimate without recourse to direct coercion. Claudius's court is a theatre of this violence: mourning hastily replaced by celebrations, crime covered by a façade of normality, and truth a scarce and dangerous commodity. Hamlet, with his unbearable emotional honesty, disturbs this fiction, becoming a threat to the established order not so much because of his actions, but because of his very existence. His mere presence disarticulates the official narrative of the court, forcing everyone to confront a reality they desperately seek to ignore.

In this context, every individual is part of a diffuse surveillance apparatus. Characters such as Polonius, Rosencrantz, and Guildenstern are not secondary figures but incarnations of the modern spy: mechanisms of control that repress dissent and monitor every word and gesture. Power, as theorised by Michel Foucault (2011) in *Surveiller et punir*, is not solely a vertical structure manifesting itself in punitive acts, but a capillary network permeating the whole society, defining the boundaries of what is permissible and speakable. The Danish court thus becomes the model of a society of control, in which individual identity is constantly under scrutiny and where truth cannot emerge freely. Hamlet, with his lucidity, opposes this system, but his resistance is not direct action; rather, it is a crisis that unfolds within language and the psyche. His feigned madness is the only possible mask to reveal the true madness of the power surrounding him, making visible the invisible structure that upholds social fiction.

In this sense, we can read Elsinore as an anticipation of modern "surveillance societies" (Lyon, 2001): a context in which power is exercised not only through visible force, but through the ability to filter and shape information flows, orienting what subjects can know, say, and believe. Claudius's figure perfectly fits into the logic of power described by Manuel Castells (2009), in which controlling the network of communications is the key to maintaining social hegemony.

The Fragmented Identity: The Modern Subject Between Doubt and Reflection

Hamlet stands at the centre of this pathological mechanism but is also the exception that reveals its cracks. He alone perceives the relationship between power, deceit, and silence, yet this awareness condemns him to profound isolation. His constant dialogue with himself, which immobilises him and postpones his action, is the symptom of a deep identity crisis. His celebrated soliloquy, *"To be or not to be"*, is not mere philosophical speculation, but the manifestation of a split identity, unable to act coherently in a world without points of reference. This impasse, which Nadia Fusini (2010) defines as the "scene of modern subjectivity", marks a radical break with classical tragedy, in which action was often driven by destiny and well-defined obligations. In *Hamlet*, the principle of action becomes a problematic question because the modern subject is required to choose in a context devoid of symbolic certainties.

From a sociological perspective, Hamlet's drama anticipates what Ulrich Beck (1992) calls "reflexive modernity", in which individuals not only live in a complex and risky world but are also compelled to reflect constantly on the very conditions of their existence. Excessive awareness does not liberate; it produces anxiety, as every choice carries irreversible consequences and no normative framework is solid enough to sustain action.

This condition foreshadows the modern subject described by Zygmunt Bauman (2000), an individual immersed in "liquid modernity", exposed to insecurity and to the responsibility of defining oneself in the absence of stable norms and lasting attachments. In a world where social structures and collective references dissolve rapidly, identity is no longer something received, but a constant individual task, laden with anxiety and ambivalence. Hamlet lives precisely this condition: he lacks a symbolic framework that could guide him unequivocally, and every choice becomes an unbearable burden, as it finds no confirmation or legitimation in a shared order.

The absence of a "communal ethos" and of a "divine law" grounding the sense of duty, as Max Weber (1995) notes in his study on the "disenchantment of the world" (*Entzauberung der Welt*), deprives Hamlet of a clear moral framework.

While classical tragedy found in divine order or the law of fate a secure anchor, the Danish prince moves in a horizon where these foundations have collapsed: avenging his father's murder is no longer an absolute duty but an insoluble ethical and psychological dilemma.

To this is added the crisis of the "Name-of-the-Father", theorised by Jacques Lacan (2008) as a central element of the symbolic structure. In *Hamlet*, the absence or corruption of this paternal function—not only the biological father but the symbolic instance guaranteeing law and the coherence of the social order—translates into a void of legitimation. Without a recognised symbolic authority, every action risks being perceived as arbitrary or illegitimate, and thus impossible to carry out fully.

In this void, alienation, in the sociological sense defined by Melvin Seeman (1959), becomes the prince's existential condition. Seeman identifies five dimensions that in Shakespeare's drama intertwine into a coherent and almost suffocating framework. Powerlessness is the first and most evident: every decision Hamlet makes seems destined to produce no concrete effect, as if the world around him were impermeable to will. Meaninglessness emerges in the question *"to be or not to be"*: the interrogation is not only metaphysical but signals a loss of meaning in the whole human experience, in which life and death appear equivalent. Anomie manifests itself in the collapse of the norms that should regulate revenge and justice: moral law is no longer univocal, and the social code is irreparably compromised by Claudius's original crime. Isolation is not only physical but above all interior: though surrounded by courtiers, Hamlet moves as a stranger in a hostile environment permeated with deceit. Finally, self-estrangement marks the most radical detachment: Hamlet no longer recognises himself in the actions he takes or in the words he utters, perceiving himself as an actor forced to play a role in a drama written by others.

This condition is aggravated by what Jan Kott (2015) recognises as the hallmark of the modern intellectual: "one who knows too much to desire naively". Knowledge does not liberate him; it imprisons him, making him a spectator of himself and of the world. Knowledge becomes an obstacle to action: every gesture is filtered through a reflection that dissects its possibilities, foresees its consequences, and relativises its necessity.

Hamlet's reflection thus does not proceed linearly towards a decision but coils upon itself, in a circular and obsessive movement that foreshadows the existential torment analysed by Søren Kierkegaard (1954) in *The Concept of Anxiety*. Here, doubt is not a stage to be overcome but a permanent condition: anxiety arises from freedom itself, from the possibility of choosing among many options without any ultimate foundation to guarantee their rightness.

In this condition of alienation and continuous reflection, Hamlet appears as a subject trapped in an inner conflict that never resolves into action. It is precisely in this suspended space, between the desire to act and the fear of consequences, that one of the most universal and elevated moments of the tragedy takes place: the "To be or not to be" soliloquy.

The "To be or not to be" Soliloquy: A Meditation on the Human Condition

The "To be or not to be" soliloquy (*Act III, Scene I*) is one of the most celebrated and quoted passages in Shakespeare's entire oeuvre, and perhaps in world literature. In just a few dozen lines, Hamlet condenses a reflection that transcends the plot's context and assumes universal value: the choice of whether to go on living or to end one's own existence. The opening question, *"to be or not to be"*, is radical because it reduces the entire human condition to an essential and definitive alternative.

The prince does not limit himself to an abstract thought on life and death: he lists the concrete reasons why life can seem unbearable—*"the slings and arrows of outrageous fortune"*—and contrasts them with the idea of rest and quiet that death might bring. Yet this attraction is immediately opposed by the fear of the unknown, *"the undiscover'd country from whose bourn no traveller returns"*. Here Shakespeare captures a universal feature of human experience: the uncertainty about what happens after death restrains many from acting against their own lives.

The soliloquy thus also becomes a discourse on fear as a conservative force: it is not will, but uncertainty, that keeps human beings in life, driving them to endure pains and injustices rather than face an obscure destiny. The image of action that "loses the name of action" because of reflection—*"thus conscience does make cowards of us all"*—opens yet another dimension: the idea that conscience and thought, though noble human qualities, can become obstacles to decision-making.

In this sense, the soliloquy is not only a personal confession but a diagnosis of the human condition in general: everyone, at some point in life, faces the conflict between the desire to end suffering and the fear of unknown consequences. The philosophical echoes are broad: from Epicurus, who urged not to fear death, to Pascal, who saw in man a fragile and restless being, up to twentieth-century existentialism, for which the freedom to choose entails the burden of deciding without certainties.

For this reason, the "To be or not to be" soliloquy continues to speak beyond eras and cultures: it is the voice of a man who, faced with the most elementary and definitive question, still chooses to interrogate himself, embodying the very act of thinking as an inescapable part of human life (Kermode, 2001).

The Social Role as Prison: Performativity and Doubt

Hamlet's tragedy is also, in a decisive way, the story of an irreconcilable conflict between subjective identity and socially imposed roles. He is, simultaneously, prince, son, avenger, Christian, intellectual—roles which in theory should form a solid identity, but which in his case overlap and contradict each other until dissolving any internal coherence. According to Robert K. Merton's (2000) theory, this condition of "role ambivalence" produces a form of paralysis: the normative expectations weighing on Hamlet—to avenge his father and, at the same time, not to commit a sin—not only diverge but mutually exclude each other. In this state, every possible action is also impossible; every choice entails the violation of a fundamental principle.

The prince thus moves in a veritable hall of mirrors, where it is no longer clear which is his authentic identity and which the role he is playing. In a pre-modern society, the role of "avenger" would have had a defined contour and an obligatory path; in Hamlet's Denmark, that role is contaminated by moral and psychological dilemmas that make it impracticable. His figure is suspended between acting and performing, between being and appearing, until the two planes merge.

In this context, social life manifests itself as a "performance", as Erving Goffman (1997) explains. Individuals, in his perspective, construct the image of themselves they wish to present to others as if on a stage, wearing masks and adapting their performance to the audience's expectations. Hamlet is not only aware of being "on stage"—he declares it, he ironises about it, he exploits it—but pushes this dynamic to the extreme when, with the "play within the play" (*The Mousetrap*), he uses artistic performance to unmask social performance. His madness, far from being a mere breakdown, functions as a conscious mask, a role constructed to destabilise the language and codes of the court.

This dualism between feigned and genuine madness, interpreted by Stephen Greenblatt (1988) as both a "survival strategy" and "an expression of an inner truth", reveals how, in Hamlet, resistance to power does not proceed through physical force but through the manipulation of language and the subversion of communicative rituals. Hamlet's speech is constantly disorienting: it alternates lyricism and sarcasm, logic and nonsense, and in so doing disrupts the communicative linearity upon which power bases its legitimacy.

Hans-Georg Gadamer (2000) has seen in *Hamlet* a drama in which truth and power collide directly: the symbolic order—the system of meanings and values that holds a community together—is destabilised by political violence and the manipulation of information. In Claudius's kingdom, the word is no longer a transparent vehicle of meaning but a weapon, an instrument for constructing and concealing reality.

Here a central knot emerges: the problem of speech. In Goffman, language is an integral part of the "staging" of social life: it serves to maintain the desired impression in the eyes of the audience. In Habermas (1981), on the other hand, speech is the foundation of the public sphere, the space in which subjects can engage in rational and free dialogue, seeking consensus that is not imposed but communicatively constructed. Hamlet, however, finds himself in a paradoxical condition: on the one hand, his speech has a revelatory potential—it can expose the truth of the crime and the hypocrisy of the court—but, on the other hand, it operates in a context where discourse is already colonised by lies and strategy, and thus every statement risks being absorbed into the fiction of power.

This tension is clearly visible in the dialogue with Rosencrantz and Guildenstern (*Act III, Scene II*), when Hamlet refuses to be "played" like a flute, accusing them of trying to manipulate him and to "pluck out the heart of my mystery": "*You would play upon me; you would seem to know my stops; you would pluck out the heart of my mystery... though you can fret me, you cannot play upon me"*. Here speech becomes an instrument of resistance: Hamlet unmasks the manipulative intent and asserts his opacity as a defence against social control.

The result is an insoluble tension: speaking is necessary to resist, but every word is vulnerable to distortion and manipulation. This condition is not merely an ethical or psychological problem but also a communicative one: Hamlet inhabits a linguistic space where speech is deprived of the capacity to transform reality, and this surprisingly anticipates the contemporary condition of language neutralised by hyper-communication and rendered harmless by its instrumental use in the media. In this sense, *Hamlet* becomes not only the tragedy of the paralysed individual but also a drama about the crisis of speech as an instrument of truth and social change.

Female Figures and Social Marginality

The figures of Ophelia and Gertrude offer another sociological lens on the drama, revealing the social marginalisation and exclusion of women within a patriarchal system. Both are trapped and subordinated to male dynamics of power. Ophelia, under the weight of social constraints and the demands of her father (Polonius), loses both her voice and her reason. Her madness is not a strategic choice but the expression of a trauma that cannot be articulated in a language of her own. Her figure, analysed by Elaine Showalter (2003), embodies female madness as social condemnation—a destiny of silence and death for those who have no place in the public discourse.

Ophelia's madness manifests itself in fragmented songs and disjointed gestures, a bodily language that replaces the speech denied to her. Her death, described in lyrical yet despairing language, symbolises the definitive exclusion of a non-conforming female subjectivity. She becomes the emblem of a culture that does not accept a woman's voice and condemns those who fail to conform to expectations of obedience and submission. Her death by drowning—merging with the natural element—is the final act of an existence taken from her, a haunting image that has inspired countless artists and interpreters.

Gertrude, on the other hand, is a character without autonomy, seen either as an object of desire or as a complicit figure, but incapable of asserting herself as a political subject. Her inability to act and to choose embodies the marginality of women within the sphere of power—a theme that makes *Hamlet* a text of profound gender sensitivity. Her role is defined entirely by her relationships with men (husband, husband's brother, son), and she never manages to impose herself as an autonomous entity. She is neither an innocent victim nor a malicious accomplice, but rather a tragic figure embodying the absence of power in a system that denies her the possibility of political subjectivity.

From the perspective of gender sociology, Ophelia and Gertrude embody what Simone de Beauvoir (1961) defined as "the Other" in the man–woman relationship:

subjects reduced to ancillary functions in a male universe, deprived of autonomous agency. The absence of authentic speech for women in the court of Elsinore is not merely a dramaturgical element, but also an index of the asymmetrical distribution of symbolic and communicative capital in a patriarchal society.

The Modernity of Hamlet: From Theatre to Cultural Resistance

The strength of *Hamlet* lies in its ability to be constantly reinterpreted, adapting to the transformations of society. Productions set in totalitarian or digital states (such as the 2025 experimental production *Hamlet: Hail to the Thief*) demonstrate how his paranoia and disorientation remain disturbingly relevant. The text becomes a tool for reflecting on pervasive surveillance, political disillusionment, and the anxiety of the contemporary world. Paranoia is no longer just a metaphor but a tangible condition in a society dominated by omnipresent technological control and the constant threat of disinformation.

Similarly, staging *Hamlet* in contexts of war and conflict (as in Aden in 2023) underscores the role of theatre as a "common good" and an act of political resistance, as UNESCO has emphasised. Bringing classical theatre to devastated cities is not only an artistic choice but an act of defiance and hope, reaffirming the value of culture as a tool of resilience. Its pedagogical dimension is crucial: *Hamlet* teaches us to ask questions, to challenge official truths, and to develop critical awareness. The personal drama of a Danish prince thus becomes a universal reflection on social structures, illusions, and the hopes of our shared humanity.

In this sense, *Hamlet* is not only a theatrical text but also what we might call a "cultural device of resistance": a narrative space in which the audience can recognise patterns of power, forms of alienation, and mechanisms of exclusion still operating in today's world. Its constant re-actualisation demonstrates theatre's capacity to function as an alternative public sphere (Fraser, 1990), in which stage dialogue opens possibilities for social critique and imagination.

Conclusion

Hamlet is not only a tragic character but a key figure for understanding modernity as a condition of disenchantment, identity instability, and social performativity. His story is that of a subject who, fully aware of the corruption of the world, finds himself paralysed by the weight of his own conscience. His inability to act is not weakness, but the representation of a profound ethical and intellectual complexity, which Yves Bonnefoy (2023) reads as a conscious refusal to "violently simplify" reality. Hamlet embodies the paradox of modern freedom: the possibility of choice is also the burden of uncertainty, and knowledge of the world does not automatically translate into the power to transform it.

If in the introduction Hamlet appeared as the forerunner of modern man, lost in a void of values, now we can also recognise him as a permanent symbol of the human struggle with uncertainty: a subject who knows, but hesitates; who speaks, but doubts the efficacy of his own words; who desires, but within roles that imprison him. This condition is not a relic of the past but a mirror of the globalised present, in which the crisis of subjectivity is fuelled by fragmented allegiances, informational overload, and the dominance of representation.

The tragedy of Hamlet is, ultimately, the tragedy of modern consciousness: a subject both aware and powerless, learned yet paralysed, who embodies the crisis of thought, desire, and memory. His failure is also his strength, for Hamlet offers no solutions but represents thought in its purest form, confronting the absence of certainties and the fracture of the self. Shakespeare's text thus remains a fertile resource not only for literary criticism but also for sociological reflection, offering a precious lens through which to analyse our world and our condition as individuals within it.

The end of the play does not resolve its problems or offer definitive answers, but rather anticipates the dilemmas of contemporary humanity and foreshadows its possible tragedies. Like Hamlet, we too are called to make a decision—whatever that decision may be.

References

Bauman, Z. (2000). *Modernità liquida*. Laterza.

Bertinetti, P. (2021). *Shakespeare Creatore di Miti, Utet.*

Bonnefoy, Y. (2023). *L'esitazione di Amleto. Scritti su William Shakespeare*. il Saggiatore.

Bourdieu, P. (2001). *La distinzione. Critica sociale del gusto*. Il Mulino.

Castells, M. (2009). *Communication power*. Oxford University Press.

De Beauvoir, S. (1961). *Il secondo sesso*. Il Saggiatore.

Foucault, M. (2011). *Storia della follia nell'età classica*. Rizzoli.

Fraser, N. (1990). Rethinking the public sphere: A contribution to the critique of actually existing democracy. *Social Text, 25*(26), 56–80.

Fusini, N. (2010). Di vita si muore. Lo spettacolo delle passioni nel teatro di Shakespeare. Mondadori

Gadamer, H.-G. (2000). *Verità e metodo*. Bompiani.

Giddens, A. (1991). *Modernity and self-identity: Self and society in the late modern age*. John Wiley and Sons.

Goffman, E. (1997). La vita quotidiana come rappresentazione. Il Mulino.

Greenblatt, S. (1988). *Shakespearean negotiations: The circulation of social energy in renaissance England*. University of California Press.

Kermode, F. (2001). Shakespeare's language. Penguin Books.

Kierkegaard, S. (1954). *Il concetto dell'angoscia*. Paravia.

Kott, J. (2015). *Shakespeare, il nostro contemporaneo*. Feltrinelli.

Lacan, J. (2008). *Il Seminario. Libro VII: L'etica della psicoanalisi*. Einaudi.

Lyon, D. (2001). *Surveillance society: Monitoring everyday life*. Open University Press.

Merton, R. K. (2000). *Teoria e struttura sociale*. Il Mulino.

Seeman, M. (1959). On the meaning of alienation. *American Sociological Review, 24*(6), 783–791.
Showalter, E. (2003). Representing Ophelia: Women, madness, and the responsibilities of feminist criticism. In *Shakespeare and the question of theory*. Methuen/Routledge.
Weber, M. (1995). Economia e società. Edizioni di comunità.

Part II
Practices

Chapter 5
Bodies, Voices, and Stories: Dramatherapy for Social and Psychological Change

Alessandro Porrovecchio

Introduction

I met her at university. She seemed beautiful to me—certainly gentle. There was something in her gaze, in the rhythm of her speech, that made me want to know her better, or at least spend time in her presence. One evening, she invited me to join a theatre group she had been attending for some months.

I felt awkward, and extremely shy. As a teenager, I had done some stand-up comedy, but that was a different world altogether. I had just begun my doctoral studies at the University of Turin, and everything around me felt new, full of possibility and uncertainty. So, I gave it a try.

I arrived late—a kind of Freudian slip, perhaps. Everyone was on their knees, arms raised, pretending to be leaves in the wind. They smiled at me, welcoming me into the exercise. It felt like a scene from an awkward 80s horror film. I lifted my arms. I became a leaf—for a very short time. Then I left.

Theatre, it seemed, was not for me. Nor was she. I had been too embarrassed. That remained my only real encounter with theatre—for years.

Until I met a student—a woman in her thirties, quietly restarting her academic path after life had taken her elsewhere for some time. She was brilliant, unusually so. Her name was Cécile. She had returned to her studies after years of life taking her back and forth across the Atlantic. We were in Calais. Her way of speaking captivated me; her ideas were vibrant and compelling. One day, looking me straight in the eyes, she said, "I am a playwright. I've just resumed my studies in adapted physical activity, and I feel a little lost. I believe these two worlds can come together", she said. And she was right, the answer was dramatherapy (DT).

A. Porrovecchio (✉)
Univ. Littoral Côte d'Opale, Univ. Lille, Univ. Artois - ULR 7369 - URePSSS - Unité de Recherche Pluridisciplinaire Sport Santé Société, Calais, France

P. Corvo, I. Riccioni (eds.), *Theatre and Quality of Life*, Social Indicators Research Series 91, https://doi.org/10.1007/978-3-032-09731-6_5

We spent a great deal of time together, caught in a virtuous whirlwind of friendship and mutual inspiration. Gradually, we began to shape our own approach to DT for social and mental health—she was the one with the vision, the expertise, and the empathy needed to lead the interventions; I observed, learned, and translated those moments into the language of research.

Our work drew on Augusto Boal's *Theatre of the Oppressed* (1979), Paulo Freire's *Pedagogy of the Oppressed* (1974), the principles of Nonviolent Communication (Rosenberg, 2002), and, most importantly, her rich experience in theatrical mediation.

Today, she is a gifted dramatherapist, working somewhere between the "here" and "there" of the Atlantic Ocean. Our brief friendship left me with cherished memories, a set of compelling ideas, and a handful of projects—some of which we developed together—that I will explore in this chapter.

This chapter is therefore structured in two parts. In the first, I introduce the concept of DT, outlining its evolution with a particular focus on Jacob Levi Moreno's psychodrama and Augusto Boal's *Theatre of the Oppressed.* In the second part, I present three ongoing projects that have each led to doctoral research initiatives. These case studies explore DT in three distinct settings: within a French Regional Special Education School (Établissement Régional d'Enseignement Adapté, EREA), which provides support to adolescents with complex educational needs; in clinical contexts with pre-bariatric patients confronting body image and self-perception; and with individuals living with rare diseases, using performative space as a means of reappropriating their embodied experience of illness.

About Dramatherapy

DT, as a distinct therapeutic approach, occupies a liminal space between psychology, sociology, and the performing arts. Over the past century, it has been shaped by a wide range of influences and traditions. Among these, the psychodrama of Jacob Levy Moreno (1987) and the *Theatre of the Oppressed* developed by Augusto Boal (1979, 1996, 2005) stand as our primary points of reference. While drama therapy shares a common genealogy with these movements, it has since evolved into a field with its own theoretical frameworks, professional standards, and therapeutic methodologies.

The Legacy of Jacob L. Moreno: From Psychodrama to Sociodrama

One of the foundational figures in the history of DT is Jacob Levy Moreno, whose contributions in the early twentieth century laid the groundwork for integrating theatrical techniques into psychotherapeutic practice. After working with socially marginalized populations in Vienna, Moreno conceived the idea of employing spontaneous dramatization as a therapeutic modality. His *Theatre of Spontaneity* (Moreno, 1987) became a platform for participants to externalize inner conflicts through improvisational performance, thus harnessing the cathartic potential of drama.

Psychodrama, as theorized by Moreno, encouraged individuals to re-enact past events, unresolved conflicts, or anticipated future situations, with the support of a group and under the direction of a trained facilitator. In this framework, the stage became both a symbolic and therapeutic space where subjective experience could be transformed into shared narrative and emotional insight (Blatner, 2000). Over time, psychodrama evolved into sociodrama, wherein the focus shifted from individual dilemmas to collective tensions. Sociodrama invited communities or groups to dramatize social issues—such as inequality, prejudice, or systemic conflict—aiming to foster group catharsis and social transformation (Karp et al., 2005). These early developments underline the dual purpose of dramatic practices: the therapeutic healing of the individual and the socio-political empowerment of the collective.

DT, while indebted to Moreno's innovations, has differentiated itself by emphasizing narrative coherence, role work, and metaphor as therapeutic tools, and by integrating insights from developmental psychology, anthropology, and psychoanalysis (Landy, 1994; Emunah, 1994).

Dramatherapy and the Theatre of the Oppressed

A second major theoretical pillar of DT derives from Augusto Boal's *Theatre of the Oppressed* (Boal, 1979, 1996, 2005), a form of applied theatre that draws explicitly on Paulo Freire's *Pedagogy of the Oppressed* (1974). Freire's notion that education should enable oppressed populations to develop critical consciousness (*conscientização*) and act as agents of social transformation profoundly influenced Boal's dramaturgical and political praxis.

In Boal's view, theatre is not a rehearsal for art, but a rehearsal for life—a space where oppressed individuals can experiment with strategies of resistance, develop alternative narratives, and challenge dominant power structures. The techniques he developed—such as *Forum Theatre*, *Image Theatre*, and *Legislative Theatre* (Boal, 1979, 2005)—were designed not for professional actors, but for everyday people, often marginalized, to become protagonists of their own struggles. Boal's concept of the "spect-actor" (spectator + actor) embodies the idea that the boundary between watching and doing can and should be broken: audiences are invited to intervene directly in the performance and propose alternative actions, thereby transforming passivity into agency (Boal, 1979, 2005; Jackson, 2007).

DT draws on these performative, dialogical, and embodied practices to empower participants, especially those experiencing social vulnerability or psychological marginalization. It offers a framework through which therapeutic change can emerge from collective engagement, emotional expression, and symbolic action. As Charbonnier (2013) emphasizes, Boal's theatre is a pedagogical and emancipatory space—a "rehearsal of revolution"—that echoes Freire's idea of the world as something that can be named and transformed through shared critical reflection (1974).

Definitions and Conceptual Grounding

Despite its increasing institutionalization, DT resists a single, universally accepted definition. The term “therapy” itself is polyvalent, and practices vary widely across cultural and clinical contexts. Nonetheless, professional associations have attempted to articulate its core principles. The North American Drama Therapy Association (NADTA) defines dramatherapy as:

> “the intentional use of drama and/or theatre processes to achieve therapeutic goals. dramatherapy is an embodied practice that is active and experiential. This approach can provide the context for participants to tell their stories, set goals and solve problems, express feelings, or achieve catharsis. Through drama, the depth and breadth of inner experience can be actively explored and interpersonal relationship skills can be enhanced [...] dramatherapy uses play, embodiment, projection, role, story, metaphor, empathy, distancing, witnessing, performance, and improvisation to help people make meaningful change” (NADTA, n.d.)

This definition highlights several central features of DT: embodiment, storytelling, role-taking, and the transformative potential of aesthetic distance. These elements enable participants to access complex emotional states, explore alternative identities, and experiment with new forms of relationality (Johnson & Emunah, 2009).

Dramatherapy and Ritual: A Liminal Framework

In recent years, scholars have increasingly emphasized the ritualistic dimensions of DT, drawing on the anthropological frameworks of Arnold van Gennep (1909), Victor Turner (1969, 1982, 1986), and Richard Schechner (1985). The therapeutic encounter is frequently structured around a liminal space, a “betwixt and between” moment in which normative roles and routines are suspended, allowing new forms of meaning-making and symbolic transformation to emerge. Turner’s notion of *communitas*—a temporary experience of egalitarian belonging generated within ritual—finds a powerful echo in the group dynamics often observed in DT sessions.

Within this perspective, the dramatic frame operates as a ritualized container for transition, a symbolic architecture in which participants can engage in embodied narratives of mourning, healing, resistance, or empowerment. Whether oriented towards psychological integration or social reconfiguration, DT mobilizes the imagination through the body—an imaginative doing that becomes a becoming, to borrow from Schechner (1985).

In my own experience—initially in collaboration with Cécile, and subsequently with other researchers involved in DT projects—what we observed over the course of the sessions, and most vividly during certain collective sequences, may be read as a ritual process. Following van Gennep’s triadic structure, one can discern three phases: separation, liminality, and reintegration. Although participants remained within the clinical setting, they appeared to gradually detach from the usual rhythms and expectations of care: bodies became activated and available, roles were loosened, language slowed down, transforming into gestures and symbols.

The liminal phase, as described by Turner, constituted a suspended moment in which the conventional identities of patient, therapist, professional, and observer became blurred. Even the simplest actions—a step, a touch, a glance—acquired an ambiguous quality, simultaneously ordinary and extraordinary. In this transitory space, the goal was not merely to do, but to become—and to become *with*. The group itself, akin to a social drama (Turner, 1986), processed latent tensions, negotiated belonging, and staged symbolic conflicts and recognitions.

Yet what occurred was not merely representation. As Schechner reminds us, ritual is performance—not a metaphor for action, but action that transforms. Performance is a becoming. The gestures we witnessed were not theatrical imitations of some distant elsewhere: they were transformative practices operating in the immediacy of the moment. Each body became simultaneously actor and witness, and through the symbolic repetition of postures, sounds, and dynamics, a dense, charged doing emerged—one capable of reconfiguring the boundaries of the pathological, the normal, and the possible.

It is from this interpretive framework that we now turn to three case studies, each illustrating different facets of this embodied, performative, and ritualized therapeutic process.

Case Studies

The ECAD Project: Dramatherapy in Special Educational Settings

This case study stems from an action-research project launched in 2021, conducted in a Special Needs Regional School (Établissement Régional d'Enseignement Adapté—EREA) in Northern France—a secondary school serving adolescents referred by regional commissions due to severe academic, social, or behavioural difficulties. Many of these students carry complex biographical trajectories marked by trauma, exclusion from mainstream education, and structural vulnerability—conditions that Gramsci (1934) might have described as being "on the margins of history".

The project was supported on two occasions by funding from the INSPE of the Académie de Lille, and was conceived and implemented in close collaboration with Cécile Nadhira Abdessemed, whose expertise in drama-based intervention played a foundational role in its development. It has so far produced an initial publication (Abdessemed & Porrovecchio, 2024) and a second article currently under review, co-authored with Bérénice Mai Pruvost, who also contributed significantly to the final phase of the fieldwork. Today, the legacy of this project continues in the form of a doctoral thesis led by Alice D'Errico in another special needs' school, with a renewed focus on the use of Boal's inspired social theatre (D'Errico & Porrovecchio, 2025) as a tool for inclusion, self-expression, and social repair among vulnerable adolescents.

An earlier investigation revealed alarming indicators: over 60% of EREA students exhibited signs of eating disorders; nearly half reported psychological distress; and high levels of sedentary behaviour and social isolation were directly correlated with risk of school disengagement. These findings prompted the research team, in collaboration with the EREA staff, to develop a series of DT workshops focused on self-expression and Boal's *Theatre of the Oppressed*.

The intervention involved three student groups from vocational training tracks: "Sanitation and Hygiene", "Agriculture", and "Landscape Gardening". A total of ten DT workshops per group were conducted, combining elements of Augusto Boal's *Theatre of the Oppressed* (Boal, 1979, 1996, 2005) with improvisation, role-playing, and bodywork. The project adopted a symbolic interactionist lens (Blumer, 1969), drawing from Goffman's (1959) theories on self-presentation and Garfinkel's (1996) ethnomethodology, aiming to reconfigure students' embodied narratives through performance.

Methodologically, the project followed Kurt Lewin's (1951) model of action-research, combining ethnographic observation (Beaud & Weber, 2003) with in-depth interviews (Kaufmann, 1996) conducted with both students and educational staff. Through this immersive qualitative approach, researchers sought to evaluate the impact of DT on students' self-perception, group belonging, and expressive capacity.

Results varied across the three groups, yet all displayed positive shifts in body language, social interaction, and verbal confidence. In the "Sanitation and Hygiene" group, initial signs of physical withdrawal and aggression gave way to more open posture and mutual respect. Among agricultural students, drama-based vocal and gestural work improved self-confidence and collective cohesion, despite lingering insecurities. The "Landscape Gardening" group showed the most pronounced progress: improved physical presence, clearer speech, and an enhanced sense of self.

Teachers' observations aligned with these findings. Several reported a transformation not only in students' behaviour but also in their own pedagogical strategies. Integrating the educators into the sessions fostered mutual understanding, allowing for more attuned and adaptive teaching approaches. Nevertheless, one group continued to display persistent internal tensions, suggesting that DT's effectiveness is also shaped by the broader classroom climate and the flexibility of pedagogical practices.

Ultimately, the project demonstrated that DT can act as a powerful tool for social and emotional rehabilitation among adolescents facing compounded forms of marginalization. By facilitating non-verbal communication, emotional literacy, and embodied self-awareness, the workshops helped reframe how students related to themselves and others. As one participant expressed: "For the first time, I didn't feel like I had to play tough—I could just breathe and be me".

Dramatherapy and Pre-Bariatric Care

The second case study, currently in its early stages, explores the integration of DT into pre- and post-operative care for patients suffering from eating disorders (EDs) and undergoing bariatric surgery. This doctoral project, funded by the Hauts-de-France Region and the University of The Littoral Opal Coast, led by the PhD candidate Suzanne Vanachter under the supervision of the present author and Professor Ariane Martinez (University of Lille), forms part of a wider collaboration between our laboratory (URePSSS—Unité de Recherche Pluridisciplinaire Sport Santé Société) and the Clinique Elsan, in Saint-Omer (France).

Eating disorders remain a major and complex public health concern in France and beyond, with prevalence figures often underestimated due to the lack of consideration of subclinical or atypical disorders (Galmiche et al., 2019). Within the bariatric population, problematic eating behaviours are particularly frequent and may significantly influence both the indication for surgery and its long-term outcomes (Conceição et al., 2015). Despite this, the integration of psychosocial interventions such as DT into the standard multidisciplinary protocol for bariatric care is still rare, and largely unexplored in the literature.

The project adopts a constructivist and interactionist framework, viewing EDs not merely as medical conditions but as socially and symbolically constructed phenomena, rooted in relational dynamics, corporeal narratives, and culturally mediated norms surrounding food, control, and embodiment. In this sense, the lived experience of patients becomes central to the therapeutic process, and DT offers a space for symbolic and embodied reappropriation of those experiences.

Building on recent evidence suggesting the benefits of arts-based therapies in the treatment of eating disorders (Bucharová et al., 2020; Wood et al., 2022), the project proposes a novel model combining DT with adapted physical activity (APA), that is

> "a cross-disciplinary body of practical and theoretical knowledge directed toward impairments, activity limitations, and participation restrictions in physical activity. It is a service delivery profession and an academic field of study that supports an attitude of acceptance of individual differences, advocates access to active lifestyles and sport, and promotes innovative and cooperative service delivery, supports, and empowerment" (IFAPA, n.d., https://ifapa.net/definition/).

While APA has proven effective in improving physical condition, body image, and mental health before and after bariatric surgery (Baillot et al., 2016; Coleman et al., 2017), its therapeutic potential may be amplified when coupled with DT, that, in this context, is not a decorative supplement but a core strategy for working on emotional expression, narrative reconstruction, and self-esteem through performative, embodied exploration.

Methodologically, the project follows a mixed-methods, experimental design, involving approximately 200 patients randomly assigned to two groups: one receiving a standard APA protocol and another participating in an APA and DT intervention. Quantitative data is collected using validated questionnaires measuring variables such as eating behaviours, emotional well-being, stress, and self-perception at multiple time points across the treatment process. In parallel, qualitative data is gathered through ethnographic fieldwork, including participant observation, semi-structured interviews, and creative tools such as identity boxes (Brown, 2018, 2019), allowing participants to express complex or difficult experiences through symbolic assemblage and storytelling.

The project is driven by a set of clearly defined objectives. These include:

- Improving the mental and social well-being of patients
- Reducing the prevalence and severity of disordered eating behaviours
- Lowering the number of patients requiring surgical intervention by enhancing pre-operative care
- Contributing to the development of a validated interdisciplinary intervention model, with broader implications for public health, mental health, and obesity care

By situating DT at the intersection of social sciences, clinical practice, and embodied creative expression, this project aspires to challenge dominant paradigms of care and to propose an alternative, human-centred model for addressing the psychological and symbolic dimensions of eating disorders in bariatric contexts.

Dramatherapy and Rare Diseases: The Myasthenia Gravis Project

The third case study explores an emerging doctoral research project focused on patients diagnosed with Myasthenia Gravis (MG), a rare neuromuscular disease characterized by fluctuating muscle weakness, fatigue, and significant psychosocial impact. The project is led by PhD candidate Célia Leclerq, under the joint supervision of neurologist Dr. Céline Tard (University Hospital, Lille) and the present author, and is funded by both the Fondation Maladies Rares and the Université du Littoral Côte d'Opale.

Despite major advances in treatment, people living with MG continue to experience diminished quality of life, often navigating between visible and invisible forms of disability. In response to this complexity, the project seeks to implement and evaluate a combined intervention of APA and DT, aiming to improve physical condition while also addressing the neglected psychological and social dimensions of the illness.

This doctoral research builds upon a 2024–2025 pilot study supported by the Fondation Maladies Rares, in memory of Mathilde Dospital. Drawing from a bio-psycho-social approach, the project is rooted in clinical sociology and embodied health research, advocating for an "ecological" model of care that considers the full spectrum of patients' lived experience.

The study design is innovative in the field of MG: a randomized cross-over trial will involve 102 patients who will take part in two intervention sequences (APA alone, then APA combined with DT, or vice versa), with evaluations at four time points (baseline, end of treatment, and follow-ups at 3 and 6 months). The two sequences will be separated by a one-year washout period, after which the intervention order will be reversed for each group. Alongside standardized questionnaires assessing fatigue, quality of life, and daily functioning, the methodology incorporates qualitative and creative tools: ethnographic observation, semi-structured interviews, focus groups, drawing, and identity boxes (Brown, 2018, 2019), which allow participants to express embodied experiences through symbolic material assemblages.

What makes this project particularly original is its focus on symbolic and corporeal reappropriation. MG often distorts the patient's relationship to their body—a body that ceases to obey, fluctuates unpredictably, and resists familiar rhythms. By integrating dramatherapy techniques—including improvisation, role play, and embodied metaphor—the intervention offers patients a performative space in which they can reframe their relationship with illness, giving voice and gesture to what is often unspeakable. This aligns with a growing body of literature highlighting the positive effects of DT in the context of neurological pathologies or their symptoms. Specifically, positive effects have been observed in patients with epilepsy (Valeta, 2017; Pinelopi et al., 2022), as well as the relevance of psychodrama for individuals living with Parkinson's disease (Zarotti et al., 2021). More broadly, DT has proven to be a valuable tool for addressing mental health challenges and supporting patients with psychiatric disorders in achieving therapeutic goals (Valeta, 2017; Pinelopi et al., 2022).

Beyond clinical outcomes, the project aims to explore deeper questions of identity, meaning, and social reintegration. How do individuals with MG redefine themselves when their sense of agency is challenged? How might collective performance allow not only for personal transformation but also for the emergence of communitas, a shared experience of vulnerability and resilience? These are the critical inquiries that dramatherapy can address, not by offering ready-made solutions, but by staging new possibilities.

Ultimately, this research aspires to develop a replicable model of care for patients with MG, demonstrating that the integration of APA and DT can generate sustained benefits in autonomy, self-perception, and quality of life. In doing so, it contributes to reframing chronic illness not only as a clinical condition, but as a relational and existential challenge—one that demands not just treatment, but meaning.

All the World's a Stage…

…and all the men and women merely players. They have their exits and their entrances, And one man in his time plays many parts" wrote William Shakespeare in *As You Like It*. This metaphor, at once poetic and deeply anthropological, continues to resonate across time. Centuries later, Erving Goffman would echo this vision, reminding us that everyday life unfolds through roles, scripts, and scenes, where the *Self* is continually performed and negotiated in interaction with others.

The three case studies presented in this chapter may differ in setting, population, and objectives. Yet they share fundamental traits that DT allows us to foreground. First, the body emerges not as an obstacle or a symptom, but as a resource: fragile, expressive, political. Second, the scene—whether improvised or structured—offers a safe and symbolic space where experiences can be externalized, reimagined, and transformed. Third, the group becomes a container of meaning, a witness and support system that allows individual narratives to emerge, circulate, and find resonance.

From a methodological perspective, each project also illuminates the challenges and tensions inherent in DT research—and in Art Based Research in general (Leavy, 2020). These include the difficulty of evaluating symbolic processes with conventional tools; the need for ethical sensitivity when engaging with vulnerable populations; and the dual position of the researcher as both observer and co-participant in the performative process. Yet it is precisely in this entanglement that rich insights are born—not despite the ambiguity, but through it.

Ultimately, these experiences invite us to reconsider care and research not as neutral, procedural domains, but as staged encounters, where gestures, silences, and presences matter as much as words. In each workshop, on each improvised stage, we catch a glimpse of what it means to become through doing, to articulate oneself not only through language but through movement, voice, and imagination.

And perhaps this is the deepest lesson of all: that if life is indeed a stage, then we must choose carefully the stories we tell, the roles we inhabit, and the spaces we create for others to perform—and to be transformed.

Acknowledgments This chapter is the result of a constellation of experiences and research projects that would not have been possible without the presence, generosity, and dedication of several individuals, as well as the support of key institutions and funding bodies.

The ECAD project was funded on two occasions by the Institut National Supérieur du Professorat et de l'Éducation (INSPE) of the Académie de Lille.

The doctoral research on pre-bariatric patients received financial support from the Région Hauts-de-France and the Université du Littoral Côte d'Opale.

The research on Myasthenia Gravis has been supported by the Fondation Maladies Rares (PhD research), in memory of Mathilde Dospital (pilot study), and by the Université du Littoral Côte d'Opale.

All these projects were supported also by the ULR 7369 URePSSS laboratory.

Special thanks go to Cécile Nadhira Abdessemed, without whom none of this would have taken shape, and to Célia Leclerq, Alice D'Errico, Suzanne Vanachter, and Bérénice Mai Pruvost for their commitment, creativity, and trust throughout each stage of these collaborative journeys.

References

Abdessemed, C. N., & Porrovecchio, A. (2024). Della drammaterapia in ambiente educativo. Un'apertura. *Corpo, Società, Educazione, 1*(0), 51–64.

Baillot, A., Mampuya, W. M., Dionne, I. J., Comeau, E., Méziat-Burdin, A., & Langlois, M. F. (2016). Impacts of supervised exercise training in addition to interdisciplinary lifestyle management in subjects awaiting bariatric surgery: A randomized controlled study. *Obesity Surgery, 26*(11), 2602–2610.

Beaud, S., & Weber, F. (2003). *Guide de l'enquête de terrain. Produire et analyser des données ethnographiques*. La découverte.

Blatner, A. (2000). *Foundations of Psychodrama: History, theory and practice* (4th ed.). Springer.

Blumer, H. (1969). *Symbolic interactionism: Perspective and method*. Berkeley.

Boal, A. (1979). *Theater of the oppressed*. Pluto Press.

Boal, A. (1996). Le 'Théâtre de l'opprimé'. *Critique communiste, 28*, 11–61.

Boal, A. (2005). *Legislative theatre: Using performance to make politics*. Routledge.

Brown, N. (2018). Identity boxes: Using material objects to elicit stories and construct meaning in qualitative interviews. *Qualitative Research, 18*(6), 656–673. https://doi.org/10.1177/1468794117741408

Brown, N. (2019). The identity box: Methodological innovations for exploring self-construction in people with chronic illness. *International Journal of Qualitative Methods, 18*, 1–12.
Bucharová, M., Malá, A., Kantor, J., & Svobodová, Z. (2020). Arts therapies interventions and their outcomes in the treatment of eating disorders: Scoping review protocol. *Behavioral Sciences, 10*(12), 188.
Charbonnier, S. (2013). À quoi reconnaît-on l'émancipation ? La familiarité contre le paternalisme. *Tracés, Revue de Sciences humaines, 25*, 83–101.
Coleman, K. J., Caparosa, S. L., Nichols, J. F., Fujioka, K., Koebnick, C., McCloskey, K. N., et al. (2017). Understanding the capacity for exercise in post-bariatric patients. *Obesity Surgery, 27*(1), 51–58.
Conceição, E. M., Utzinger, L. M., & Pisetsky, E. M. (2015). Eating disorders and problematic eating behaviours before and after bariatric surgery: Characterization, assessment and association with treatment outcomes. *European Eating Disorders Review, 23*(6), 417–425.
D'Errico, A., & Porrovecchio, A. (2025). Le Teatro Sociale en contexte éducatif en Italie. *EMPAN. Prendre la mesure à l'humain, 138*, 121–128.
Emunah, R. (1994). *Acting for real: Drama therapy process, technique, and performance*. Brunner/Mazel.
Freire, P. (1974). *Pedagogia do Oprimido*. Editora Paz e Terra.
Galmiche, M., Déchelotte, P., Lambert, G., & Tavolacci, M. P. (2019). Prevalence of eating disorders over the 2000–2018 period: A systematic literature review. *The American Journal of Clinical Nutrition, 109*(5), 1402–1413.
Garfinkel, H. (1996). Ethnomethodology's program. *Social Psychology Quarterly, 59*(1), 5–21.
Goffman, E. (1959). *The presentation of self in everyday life*. Doubleday.
Gramsci, A. (1934). Ai margini della storia (storia dei gruppi sociali subalterni). *Quaderni del carcere, 4*, 2277–2307.
Jackson, A. (2007). *Theatre, education and the making of meanings: Art or instrument?* Manchester University Press.
Johnson, D. R., & Emunah, R. (2009). *Current approaches in drama therapy*. Charles C Thomas.
Karp, M., Holmes, P., & Tauvon, K. B. (2005). *The handbook of psychodrama*. Routledge.
Kaufmann, J. C. (1996). *L'entretien compréhensif*. Nathan.
Landy, R. J. (1994). *Drama therapy: Concepts, theories and practices*. Charles C Thomas.
Leavy, P. (2020). *Method meets art: Arts-based research practice*. Guilford Publications.
Lewin, K. (1951). *Field theory in social science: Selected theoretical papers*. Cartwright.
Moreno, J. L. (1987). *The essential Moreno: Writings on psychodrama, group method, and spontaneity*. Springer Publishing Company.
Pinelopi, V., Aikaterini, T., Anna, T., Alexandrina, N., Theofanis, V., Konstantinos, V., & Ioannis, H. (2022). Changes in the quality of life of persons with epilepsy, after the implementation of an occupational therapy intervention with drama activities. *Epilepsy & Behavior, 130*, 108694.
Rosenberg, M. B. (2002). *Nonviolent communication: A language of compassion*. Puddledancer press.
Schechner, R. (1985). *Between theater & anthropology*. University of Pennsylvania Press.
Turner, V. (1969). *The ritual process. Structure and anti-structure*. Aldine Transaction.
Turner, V. (1982). *From ritual to theater: The human seriousness of play*. PAJ Publications.
Turner, V. (1986). *The anthropology of performance*. PAJ Publications.
Valeta, T. (2017). Psychological treatments for epilepsy. In *The Epilepsy book: A companion for patients: Optimizing diagnosis and treatment* (pp. 119–126).
Van Gennep, A. (1909). *Les rites de passage*. É. Nourry.
Wood, L. L., Hartung, S., Al-Qadfan, F., Wichmann, S., Cho, A. B., & Bryant, D. (2022). Drama therapy and the treatment of eating disorders: Advancing towards clinical guidelines. *The Arts in Psychotherapy, 80*, 101948.
Zarotti, N., Eccles, F. J., Foley, J. A., Paget, A., Gunn, S., Leroi, I., & Simpson, J. (2021). Psychological interventions for people with Parkinson's disease in the early 2020s: Where do we stand? *Psychology and Psychotherapy: Theory, Research and Practice, 94*(3), 760–797.

Chapter 6
Theatre, Violence, and Collective Memory

Ulrike Loch

Introduction

Maurice Halbwachs (1941/1992) drew the attention of sociological research to collective memory, which he understands as the construction of the past for the realisation of the present life. Collective memory, which is constructed through space, rites, symbols, myths, written documents, and narratives, is particularly relevant for the production of identity and belonging within social groups. Aleida Assmann (2018, p. 13) subdivides collective memory into cultural and communicative memory, with the latter considered oral memory, whose contents are passed on orally within three generations via stories, narrations, or latent transmissions, such as silence.

Sociological biographical research and oral history have shown—through narrative analysis—the close relationship between collective/personal memory and the development of people's social identity. Biographical case reconstructions show the challenges people take on to construct identity-forming life narrations that enable social belonging (Fischer-Rosenthal, 1995; Rosenthal, 2010), as well as the close connections between the failure of a biographical narrative, and social alienation and psychiatric illnesses (Riemann, 1987; Schulze, 2006). In her trauma-theoretical research, Rosenthal (1995, 1998/2010) discusses the healing effect of biographical narrations and the relevance of silence in the context of communicative memory. This entails that collective and personal memory are viewed as strongly interconnected (Duling, 2011); for Maurice Halbwachs (1941/1992), human memory cannot function without society. In addition, well-being and the success of socially accepted biographical narratives are closely linked.

U. Loch (✉)
Free University of Bolzano-Bozen, Bolzano, BZ, Italy
e-mail: Ulrike.Loch@unibz.it

P. Corvo, I. Riccioni (eds.), *Theatre and Quality of Life*, Social Indicators Research Series 91, https://doi.org/10.1007/978-3-032-09731-6_6

Sieder (1999) describes the relationship between personal and collective memory as both working in the present and constructing connections in the dimensions of time and space, developments, and origins to legitimise the present and design the future (p. 234). The relationship between the two memories significantly influences people's self-construction and their social inclusion. Moreover, Sieder maintains that collective and personal identities are relational (p. 235). As a result, new cultures of remembrance—expressed, for example, in new narratives in literature and theatre and their reception—(can) change collective memory and thus enable other biographical narrations.

Ambivalences and even conflicts between the need to speak and remaining silent can be observed in European societies in recent decades concerning the topic of sexual violence against children and adolescents. Social power is expressed in this collective silence, because silence helps perpetrators in particular, while victims need the social acknowledgement of the violent acts they have suffered (cf. Assmann, 2006; Herman, 1992/2022). Based on Aleida Assmann's work, Meike Baader (2024) emphasises that scientific power, too, has silenced violence in educational institutions for decades.

The following sections will show how theatre can contribute to incorporating the perspectives of victims in societal discussions about violence against children and adolescents and thus to updating communicative and cultural memory. Enabling former victims to talk about their suffering returns their social credibility to them, and thus contributes to their well-being.

This is shown by the study on "Gewalt an Kärntner Kindern und Jugendlichen in Institutionen" (2016–2021; Loch et al., 2022)[1] and the theatre play "Nicht sehen" (Brusilovsky, 2022) and their social and political framing. Prior to illustrating the study, the article will briefly refer to groundbreaking international and national developments that have contributed to changing perspectives in the context of violence against children and adolescents.

Societal Background

Since the year 2000, European societies have increasingly and inevitably been confronted with the disclosure of (sexualised) violence against children and young people in their social, health, and education systems by the victims and the media. In response to these revelations, initially in Ireland, commissions have been set up and ombudspersons designated in many European countries and regions, with their work often supported by research projects.

[1] The research was funded by Ärztekammer für Kärnten, KABEG/Klinikum Klagenfurt, Kärnten Privatstiftung, Province Carinthia, Österreichische Gesellschaft für Kinder- und Jugendpsychiatrie, Psychosomatik und Psychotherapie (ÖGKJP), Universität Klagenfurt as well as by private donors and enterprises.

These historical reappraisals have happened in the knowledge that social confrontation with violence in institutions such as residential care services or hospitals is a prerequisite for sustainable violence prevention. This is the case even if each confrontation is painful for the people formerly affected by violence (victims), for the (former) employees of these institutions, for the current management of the affected institutions, and for wider society. Indeed, the causes of pain and other strong emotions such as shame when confronted with sexual violence differ according to, for example, whether a person suffered from this violence or was involved as a perpetrator in acts of violence, or as a witness who covered up violent acts.[2] Nevertheless, at societal levels, there is no alternative to this harmful confrontation with violent pasts for developing a democratic future, as shown by research (Unabhängige Kommission, 2020). Investigations have been conducted in most European countries. For example, North Ireland documented, in the Historical Institutional Abuse Inquiry (Hart et al., 2017), violence against children and young people in institutions which provided residential care for children from 1922 to 1995 (including hospitals, juvenile justice institutions, denominational institutions, and institutions under local authorities). Another example is the report of the Independent Commission on sexual violence in the catholic church in France (CIASE, 2021) between the years 1950 and 2000.

In Austria, the child and youth welfare system is strongly regionally structured. Therefore, ombudspersons who monitor children's and young people's well-being have mainly regional responsibilities that are often limited regarding the examined institutions because they are mostly financed by organisations such as dioceses, monasteries, or welfare agencies. This strong regional or organisational orientation also influences research funding (Sting, 2011). Consequently, many regional research studies have been conducted in Austria since 2010, when the first cases of sexual violence in child and youth (welfare) institutions received public and media attention linked to the international reappraisal of violence in institutions.[3]

Collaboration Between Experts in the Field and Research

Following this Austrian policy, in 2013, the first Carinthian ombuds commission (2013–2015) was installed by the provincial government to offer support to victims of violence in Landesjugendheim Rosental, a sizeable residential care institution for male children and youngsters, and in the Heilpädagogische Abteilung, the

---

[2] For the social significance of secrets and secret-keepers, see Simmel (1906/2010), and in reference to this Loch et al. (2022, pp. 350–356).

[3] For Austrian studies about violence in child and youth placement, see, for example, Helige et al. (2013) for Vienna and Ralser et al. (2017) for Tyrol and Vorarlberg. For therapeutic pedagogic institutions, see, for example, Friedmann (2022) and Medizinische Universität (MedUni] Wien (2011) for Vienna or the Medizin-Historische ExpertInnenkommission (2013) for Innsbruck. For Carinthien, see Elezović et al. (2017), Imširović et a. (2019) or Loch et al. (2022).

therapeutic pedagogic[4] department of the hospital Landeskrankenhauses in Klagenfurt. This hospital department was a forerunner of today's child and youth psychiatry. The narrations of the victims in both institutions document different kinds of systemic violence, with an overwhelming majority of sexual violence in the context of medical examinations (Liebhauser, 2017). This means that, in the first years of the commission, more than 100 victims testified to various forms of violence in different provincial institutions whose societal and legal task was to support children and adolescents by offering care, healthcare, and education.

The main perpetrator accused by the victims was the respected paediatrician Franz Wurst, professor at the University of Vienna. He was the chief physician of the therapeutic pedagogic department of the hospital Landeskrankenhaus Klagenfurt, and a celebrated multi-award-winning doctor styled "Child's lawyer" in an encomium in 2000. A few months later, he was arrested and, in 2002, convicted of sexual abuse of children and adolescents under protection, among other crimes. In the following years, his conviction was ignored by the hospital management, provincial administration, and the government, as well as by socially influential associations such as the Carinthian Medical Association and by other relevant societal actors such as the Freemasons, with the result that public talk about this crime was silenced and remained taboo.

In 2015, the independent Carinthian ombudsperson's reflections became the starting point for a steering group (consisting of experts from the field, an ombudsperson, and a researcher) that explored the social consequences of documented violence. This collaboration led to the research project "Violence against Carinthian Children and Young People in Institutions" (2016–2021) (Imširović et al. (2019); Loch et al., 2022).

Since both the data from the ombuds commission and the research results clearly show the systemic failures in (social and public health) politics and administrations and organisations tasked with caring for, healing, educating, and directly supporting children and young people, questions about social consequences arose. What should be inferred from the knowledge about the failures of the helping systems? How can the results be communicated and shared outside scientific publishing? How can we use the research results to support the former victims of these systems in gaining social recognition by breaking the silence and thus increasing their well-being? Given the high number of victims as well as families affected by violence, these questions have become important for the steering group; that is where literature, theatre, and political acting joined the discussion, thus informing the study here reported. The research design will be briefly described before exploring the societal role of theatre in greater depth.

[4] Since the 1930s, the main representatives of the Austrian therapeutic pedagogy tradition are Franz Hamburger, Hans Asperger, and Franz Wurst. Hamburger and Asperger increased the alignment of therapeutic pedagogy with National Socialist ideology and system (Medizinische Universität Wien (MedUni Wien), 2011; Czech, 2018). Therapeutic pedagogies also blamed the victims of sexual violence from the inception of this discipline (Friedmann, 2022).

Research Design

The study adopts a multi-level approach. On the one hand, the case files of the Independent Carinthian Ombuds Commission were hermeneutically analysed with the consent of the former victims who had turned to the ombudspersons. On the other, 90 semi-structured interviews were conducted with professionals from various groups, scientists, and people formerly affected by violence, and also hermeneutically analysed. In addition, research was carried out in various archives, mostly in Austria. Finally, the empirical results of the respective data categories (e.g. interviews, etc.) were triangulated and related to other content-relevant theories and empirical research (cf. Loch et al., 2022, pp. 37–41).

The central research questions were: What institutional and social structures made possible the decades of violence against children and adolescents in the context of provincial therapeutic pedagogical institutions? What part did science play in maintaining violence? What insights can be gained from the study for future developments in child protection, child and youth welfare, and child and adolescent psychiatry?

The research was supported by the previously mentioned steering group. This group was primarily engaged in the historical contextualisation of the research, access to data, and the communication of the research results to professionals and the public.

Communication of the Research Results and Their Reception

From the beginning of the study, there was broad public interest in the results, reflected, among other things, in many (informal) requests for interim results. Moreover, from the start, the researchers' actions were constantly scrutinised, particularly by people formerly affected by violence, and discussed controversially in their forums, as such people later told the researchers. Through fear of disappointment, the forum discussions focused on questions such as the trustworthiness of the researchers and the independence of the research. Once trust in the autonomy of the study was achieved, former victims of violence asked for greater involvement in the study. This was expressed in their great willingness to be interviewed, even though they knew by experience about the burden of memories during and after interviews. Indeed, their explicit intention was to contribute to preventing violence against children and young people so that they would not suffer the same pain and social isolation from the violence that the study participants had experienced and continued to experience when they raised the issue socially. In addition to research, some of them also called for public discussion so as to be free of the stigma linked to having received psychiatric treatment in childhood or being a careleaver, as well as of the consequences of experiencing violence, for example, alcohol addiction or repeated relationship breakdowns.

The encounters with interviewees who still suffer from the stress of violence in out-of-home care and the documented violence in the files of the ombuds commission resulted in a wish as well as a perceived ethical obligation, on the part of researchers, to seek for opportunities to initiate a public discussion of the research results. Accordingly, a search was initiated for socially influential cultural and political spaces and collaboration partners who could enable research-informed social discourses about violence against children and young people, with the aim of dismantling the secrets and silence that surround sexual violence and abuse of power in clinical contexts.

This search led to cooperating with the Carinthian government and the Klagenfurt theatre, resulting in the following events:

Political Act

In the provincial act "Gesture of Responsibility" (2022), the Carinthian governor took political responsibility for the violence and failure of the public health and social system from 1950 to 2000, apologising to people formerly affected by violence. This political recognition of injustice has supported individual and collective healing, as an encouragement to break the taboo and view institutional violence from the perspective of those affected. This was integrated into a presentation of the research results, which, in terms of language and content, was aimed at people who mostly knew the content from their life experiences. In this context, social sciences took on the task of "voicing" (cf. Hirschauer, 2001, p. 438), i.e., verbalising the injustice in the presence of those formerly directly affected by violence, so that experiences acquired public social and political relevance. This was reinforced by reading the literary text "Kindermund" through which the writer Anna Baar (2022) embedded institutional violence in cultural memory. The reading was accompanied by podcasts in which people who had previously been affected by violence had their say, with dignity and anonymously. It was a symbolic event, significantly held in a public building (the concert hall of the provincial capital) where the traumatic life experiences of the former victims became manifested in a language that transferred those experiences into the collective past. Every participant was thus conscious of the significance of this historical moment.

Theatre Play

The theatre director Noam Brusilovsky (2022) and his team developed the play "Nicht sehen" with a participatory approach based on the main project publication "Im Namen von Wissenschaft und Kindeswohl" (Loch et al., 2022), and their own research. Due to the participatory approach, the theatre project included Carinthian citizens as actors and contemporary witnesses, a youth theatre group, and professional actors. Additionally, it adopted locational references such as the Landesjugendheim Rosental and the villa formerly belonging to the therapeutic pedagogic couple Hilde and Franz Wurst—together with other former party places for bourgeois society, politicians, and scientists—so as to involve the theatregoers emotionally.

The reception of the play took place both in a moderated sphere within the theatre (in particular, through audience discussions after each production) and outside, for example, in the daily press and on social media as well as in diverse societal spaces and in private communication, as evidenced from emails to researchers among other communications. Those involved in the reception (both inside and outside) included people who had been personally affected by violence in childhood and youth, their family members, former colleagues of the perpetrators, scientists, bio-psycho-social experts, socio-political actors, and previously uninvolved theatregoers. The actors also expressed on stage their own confrontation with the injustice that prompted the theatre project. Thus, theatre enabled the play to be received by members of different generations. The discussion generated controversy, especially between elderly people with knowledge of the taboo and parts of its content, and younger generations who demanded an outright social repudiation of the trivialisation of the historical violence against children. Furthermore, the non-directly involved younger generations demanded to take over social responsibility. Theatre thus became "a place for interception, response and organization of collective needs" (Riccioni, 2023, p. 20)—a space where public opinion develops, and topics can be revisited based on what is presented and its reception.

Thanks to a range of elements and strategies, including: the broad social reception of the play "Nicht sehen" and the literary text "Kindermund", the broad participation in the political act by the affected people, their relatives and politicians, the wide dissemination of the research publications, and the conferences primarily aimed at bio-psycho-social professionals, the perspective of people formerly directly affected by violence has now become part of the collective memory in Carinthia/Austria.[5] The collective memory has thus shifted from a perpetrator-oriented silence to one that is hospitable and able to listen to the victims of violence. As a consequence, social changes and inclusion have been requested in public.

[5] Kindermund was immediately published in the national daily press; Anna Baar has taken up the topic of silencing in many publications (https://annabaar.at/literatur.html), in 2022, she was awarded the "Großer Österreichischer Staatspreis", the highest cultural award in the Austrian Republic. Noam Brusilovsky received the award "Nestroy Preis" (2022), the most important award for theatre in Austria, for "Nicht sehen" (https://www.noam-brusilovsky.com). Ulrike Loch was awarded with the "Kärntner Menschenrechtspreis" (2019) for the presented research project. Also, these awards express cultural and collective memory changes in Austria and internationally. See for example the blog "Im Namen von Wissenschaft und Kindeswohl: Buchpublikation und Theaterstück zur Gewalt an Kindern und Jugendlichen in heilpädagogischen Institutionen der Jugendwohlfahrt und des Gesundheitswesens in Kärnten zwischen 1950 und 2000 – Universität Klagenfurt" (accessed online: 29.11.2025).

Theatre, Collective Memory, and Well-being

In the example presented, theatre was made available as a space for the social processing of the collective (cultural and communicative) memory of violence in institutions. It thus became a place for encountering, listening and understanding, reflection, contradiction, and conciliatory dialogue, which has continued in other social circles, institutions, and spaces.

This was possible because theatre aptly confronted the past violence that had taken place in Carianthia by listening to the stories of former victims of violence and afterwards incorporating their stories into a play. This methodological approach corresponds to the international studies cited at the beginning. Regret without a concrete historical or biographical reference, formulated in platitudes such as "Terrible what happened back then" or "Children should never again be harmed", has no lasting effect on changing attitudes or collective memories, as previous research on child protection shows. Coming to terms with violence as a contribution to inclusion and the development of democratic society requires reflection on concrete historical violence from the perspectives of the victims in connection with human rights-oriented actions (Unabhängige Kommission, 2020).

Which social impact has been observed after the confrontation with historical violence in the theatre?

- Theatre made it easier for families to confront the shameful secret of the out-of-home placement of a family member. In an audience discussion (after the play), for example, a man reported that only in the theatre had he learnt from his mother that his father was a victim of violence such as that depicted in the play. He reported his shock at having been excluded from such an important part of his family history, as well as his new understanding of various reactions on the part of his parents. These research results thus indicate that such situations are painful, but that they foster new relationship qualities within families.
- Secrets such as the massive suffering inflicted by violence are conveyed transgenerationally in a latent way (Rosenthal, 1998/2010; Loch, 2006). They create rifts between the knowing and the ignorant family members, even if the violence suffered was not communicated to children or grandchildren so as to protect them (i.e. with the best of intentions). Transgenerational family dialogues about violence can have a liberating effect for all generations if they take place in a socially supportive setting. Moreover, they affect the communicative memory that influences the well-being of human beings.
- Everyone involved in the theatre play has changed their understanding of violence through the participatory production, which was oriented towards the perspective of the victims of violence. One member of the youth theatre said in the audience discussion that she had learned that violence begins with the acceptance of exclusion.
- Theatre, as a medium for dealing with collective narratives, has the creative power to transform the collective construction of history through the audience's reception. If theatre develops cultural narratives that can overcome previous

norms, such as silencing violence, that achieves a change in cultural memory. As the construction of collective and personal memory is interconnected, this also influences the biographical narrations of the former victims of violence and thus their social inclusion.

- In the context of recognising violence as an injustice, theatre and other social and political actors can have an inclusive effect on people who have so far been excluded, and evoke resistance and/or reflection in those who benefit from concealing acts of violence.

To summarise, theatre can greatly influence the construction of violence in cultural and communicative memory if society accepts it and receives the acts. Naming historical violence as injustice has far-reaching effects on the social positioning of victims and influences their current well-being and the democratic development of society.

References

Assmann, A. (2006). *Der lange Schatten der Vergangenheit. Erinnerungskultur und Geschichtspolitik*. Beck. https://doi.org/10.17104/9783406622625-272

Assmann, A. (2018). *Erinnerungsräume. Formen und Wandlungen des kulturellen Gedächtnisses*. Beck. https://doi.org/10.17104/9783406729911

Baader, M. (2024). Vom beredten Schweigen der Disziplin Erziehungswissenschaft im Umgang mit sexualisierter Gewalt in Geschichte und Gegenwart. *Erziehungswissenschaft, 35*(1, 68), 15–26. https://doi.org/10.3224/ezw.v35i1.03

Baar, A. (2022). Kindermund. In U. Loch, E. Imširović, J. Arztmann, & I. Lippitz (Eds.), *Im Namen von Wissenschaft und Kindeswohl. Gewalt an Kindern und Jugendlichen in heilpädagogischen Institutionen der Jugendwohlfahrt und des Gesundheitswesens in Kärnten zwischen 1950 und 2000* (pp. 13–16). Studienverlag.

Brusilovsky, N. (2022). *Nicht sehen*. Retrieved July 11, 2024, from https://www.noam-brusilovsky.com/nicht-sehen.

CIASE (Commission indépendante sur les abus sexuels dans l'Église). (2021). *Les violences sexuelles dans l'Église catholique France 1950–2020*. CIASE.

Czech, H. (2018). Hans Asperger, National Socialism, and 'race hygiene' in Nazi-era Vienna. *Molecular Autismn, 9*(1), art. 29. https://doi.org/10.1186/s13229-018-0208-6

Duling, D. (2011). Memory, collective memory, orality and the gospels. *HTS Theological Studies, 67*(1) art. 915. https://doi.org/10.4102/hts.v67i1.915

Elezović, A., Lippitz, I., & Loch, U. (2017). Heilpädagogische Diagnostik. Zur wissenschaftlichen Stigmatisierung von Kindern und Jugendlichen, die an den Folgen von sexualisierter Gewalt litten. *Erziehungswissenschaft, 28*(1, 54), 63–74. https://doi.org/10.3224/ezw.v28i1.08

Fischer-Rosenthal, W. (1995). Schweigen—Rechtfertigen—Umschreiben. Biographische Arbeit im Umgang mit deutschen Vergangenheiten. In P. Alheit & W. Fischer-Rosenthal (Eds.), *Biographien in Deutschland. Soziologische Rekonstruktionen gelebter Gesellschaftsgeschichte* (pp. 43–86). Westdeutscher Verlag. https://doi.org/10.1007/978-3-663-09434-0_3

Friedmann, I. (2022). Abnormalität (de-)konstruiert. Die Heilpädagogische Abteilung der Wiener Universitäts-Kinderklinik und ihre Patient*innen in der ersten Hälfte des 20. Jahrhunderts. Böhlau. https://doi.org/10.7767/9783205215431.

Halbwachs, M. (1941/1992). *On collective memory* [La topographie légendaire des évangiles en terre sainte. Étude de mémoire collective] (L. A. Coser, transl., The heritage of sociology). Chicago University Press (French original work published 1941).
Hart, A., Doherty, G., & Lane, D. (2017). Historical institutional abuse inquiry. HIA. Retrieved July 11, 2024, from https://www.hiainquiry.org/historical-institutional-abuse-inquiry-report-chapters.
Helige, B., John, M., Schmucker, H., & Wörgötter, G. (2013). Endbericht der Kommission Wilhelminenberg. University of Vienna. Retrieved July 11, 2024, from http://www.kommission-wilhelminenberg.at/presse/jun2013/Bericht-Wilhelminenberg-web_code.pdf.
Herman, J. L. (1992/2022). Trauma and recovery. The aftermath of violence—from domestic abuse to political terror (4th ed). Basic Books. Original work published 1992.
Hirschauer, S. (2001). Ethnografisches Schreiben und die Schweigsamkeit des Sozialen. Zu einer Methodologie der Beschreibung. *Zeitschrift für Soziologie, 30*(6), 429–451. https://doi.org/10.1515/zfsoz-2001-0602
Imširović, E., Lippitz, I., & Loch, U. (2019). Totale Institutionalisierung als Gewalt an Kindern und Jugendlichen. *Österreichisches Jahrbuch für Soziale Arbeit, 1*(1), 49–76. https://doi.org/10.30424/OEJS1901049
Liebhauser, A. (2017). Bericht über die Tätigkeit der Opferschutzstelle und Opferschutzkommission des Landes Kärnten von Dezember 2013 bis Dezember 2015, aktualisiert mit Inkrafttreten des Heimopferrentengesetzes mit 1.7.2017.
Loch, U. (2006). *Sexualisierte Gewalt in Kriegs- und Nachkriegskindheiten. Lebens- und familiengeschichtliche Verläufe (Rekonstruktive Forschung in der Sozialen Arbeit, Vol. 2).* Budrich. https://doi.org/10.2307/j.ctvbkjtfs
Loch, U., Imširović, E., Arztmann, J., & Lippitz, I. (2022). *Im Namen von Wissenschaft und Kindeswohl. Gewalt an Kindern und Jugendlichen in heilpädagogischen Institutionen der Jugendwohlfahrt und des Gesundheitswesens in Kärnten zwischen 1950 und 2000.* Studienverlag.
Medizin-Historische ExpertInnenkommission. (2013). Die Innsbrucker Kinderbeobachtungsstation von Maria Nowak-Vogl. *Bericht.* Medizinische Universität Innsbruck. Retrieved July 11, 2024, from https://www.i-med.ac.at/pr/presse/2013/Bericht-Medizin-Historische-ExpertInnenkommission_2013.pdf
Medizinische Universität Wien (MedUni Wien). (2011). *Chronik der Universitäts-Kinderklinik Wien.* MedUni Wien.
Ralser, M., Bischoff, N., Guerrini, F., Jost, C., Leitner, U., & Reiterer, M. (2017). *Heimkindheiten. Geschichte der Jugendfürsorge und Heimerziehung in Tirol und Vorarlberg*. Studienverlag.
Riccioni, I. (2023). The social and political impact of the theatre in contemporary society. In I. Riccioni (Ed.), *Theatre(s) and public sphere in a global and digital society. Vol. 1: Theoretical explanations (studies in critical social sciences, Vol. 235; pp. 16–40).* Brill. https://doi.org/10.1163/9789004529816_003
Riemann, G. (1987). *Das Fremdwerden der eigenen Biographie. Narrative Interviews mit psychiatrischen Patienten (Übergänge, Vol. 19).* Fink. https://doi.org/10.30965/9783846723968
Rosenthal, G. (1995). Erlebte und erzählte Lebensgeschichte. Gestalt und Struktur biographischer Selbstbeschreibungen. Campus.
Rosenthal, G. (Ed.). (1998/2010). *The Holocaust in three generations. Families of victims and perpetrators of the Nazi regime* 2nd rev ed. Budrich. Original work published 1998. https://doi.org/10.2307/j.ctvddzxt6
Schulze, H. (2006). *Migrieren—Arbeiten—Krankwerden. Eine biographietheoretische Untersuchung (Kultur und soziale Praxis).* Transcript. https://doi.org/10.14361/9783839404959
Sieder, R. (1999). Gesellschaft und Person: Geschichte und Biographie. Nachschrift. In R. Sieder (Ed.), *Brüchiges Leben. Biographien in sozialen Systemen (Kultur als Praxis, Vol. 1; pp. 234–264).* Turia + Kant.
Simmel, G. (1906/2010). The sociology of secrecy and of secret societies. In G. Simmel, Gesamtausgabe. Vol. 18: Englischsprachige Veröffentlichungen 1893-1910 (pp. 405–462). Suhrkamp (Original work published 1906).

Sting, S. (2011). Disziplin, meine Damen und Herren! In M. Anastasiadis, A. Heimgartner, H. Kittl-Satran, & M. Wrentschur (Eds.), *Sozialpädagogisches Wirken (Soziale Arbeit—Social Issues, Vol. 13; pp. 36–55)*. Lit.

Unabhängige Kommission zur Aufarbeitung sexuellen Kindesmissbrauchs. (2020). *Rechte und Pflichten: Aufarbeitungsprozesse in Institutionen. Empfehlungen zur Aufarbeitung sexuellen Kindesmissbrauchs* (Geschichten, die zählen). Unabhängige Kommission. Retrieved July 11, 2024, from https://www.aufarbeitungskommission.de/wp-content/uploads/Empfehlungen-Aufarbeitung-sexuellen-Kindesmissbauchs_Aufarbeitungskommission-2020.pdf

Chapter 7
Setting the Stage: Unlocking Future Skills in the Performing Arts Sector

Moreno Zago

Cultural and Creative Industries

The concept of 'cultural industry' was initially introduced by Adorno & Horkheimer (1947/2002) within their critical examination of mass culture and consumer society. Their seminal work, 'Dialectic of Enlightenment', presented the idea that cultural production under capitalism leads to commodification, standardization, and homogenization. According to them, cultural goods—including music, cinema, literature, and theatre—are mass-produced, conforming to formulaic patterns primarily designed to maximize profit, rather than promote genuine artistic creativity or cultural enrichment. They critically argued that such standardization contributes to cultural impoverishment, limiting critical thinking among audiences and perpetuating consumer passivity.

Such standardization was interpreted as a mechanism of ideological control, reducing diversity of expression and promoting conformity through standardized mass-market cultural products.

Following the original theorization by Adorno & Horkheimer, subsequent scholars have elaborated and complicated the notion by a considerable degree. The very terms evolved into the plural 'cultural industries' to acknowledge the diversity, complexity, and dynamism within the sector. Hesmondhalgh (2019), for example, builds on this notion by highlighting the multifaceted interplay between creativity, cultural expression, technological innovation, and economic structures. Through his expansive work, he illustrates how cultural and creative industries extend beyond a purely commercial logic, engaging with issues of identity formation, social cohesion, power relations, and meaning making in profound ways.

M. Zago (✉)
University of Trieste, Trieste, TS, Italy
e-mail: MORENO.ZAGO@dispes.units.it

P. Corvo, I. Riccioni (eds.), *Theatre and Quality of Life*, Social Indicators Research Series 91, https://doi.org/10.1007/978-3-032-09731-6_7

Furthermore, the notion of 'creative industries', popularized by Florida (2002, 2012) represents a significant advancement. This approach places creativity and innovation at the centre of economic growth strategies, recognizing that cultural production extends beyond the arts to encompass design, architecture, media, digital technologies, etc. The creative economy, as Florida argues, harnesses cultural capital, talent attraction, and innovation to stimulate urban and regional regeneration, thereby shaping decisions related to policymaking worldwide, at both the national and local levels. His argument emphasizes how the attraction and fostering of a 'creative class' has rapidly become an important goal for policymakers trying to promote urban development and economic sustainability. As Santagata (2009) argues, cultural and creative sectors are not simply powerful drivers of economic growth but can function as particularly potent catalysts for economic revitalization that foster regional competitiveness, employment opportunities, and identity/belonging-driven community development. The intersection between cultural value and economic value positions these industries very well to address contemporary social challenges—particularly within urban environments.

In expanding on these ideas further, the sociological studies recognize how cultural and creative industries each not only occupy economic space but also gain social and symbolic importance. Cultural products convey meanings, shape identities, both perpetuate and reflect social norms, and serve as mechanisms for social integration and community cohesion. Theatre, literature, film, music, and other art forms create models of cultural dialogue, provoke critical reflection about societal issues, and often simultaneously work towards community building and social cohesion (Belfiore & Bennett, 2008; Boccella & Salerno, 2017).

The European Union has identified creative and cultural industries as a priority ecosystem for the single market, particularly recognizing their role in innovation and internationalization (De Voldere et al., 2017; European Commission, 2021; Pignatti, 2021, Vilares et al., 2022). Current EU programmes (2021–2027) such as 'Creative Europe' and 'Horizon' Europe specifically aim to support cultural creators and enterprises, encouraging innovative research, job creation, improved competitiveness, and fostering synergies between businesses and research institutions. These programmes also integrate environmental sustainability and social inclusion objectives outlined in the European Green Deal and the UN's Agenda 2030. Another significant European initiative mentioned is the 'New European Bauhaus', which combines art, culture, science, and technology to address contemporary urban planning challenges, sustainability, and accessibility by reinterpreting Europe's cultural heritage. At the European level, cultural and creative industries contribute significantly to the economy, accounting for over 4% of the European Union's GDP and providing employment for approximately nine million people (Symbola, 2024: 27).

Creative labour itself has become a critical object of sociological inquiry. The sociological literature emphasizes how creative professionals face increasingly precarious working conditions, characterized by freelance or project-based employment, short-term contracts, low job security, and unpredictable income streams. Creative work often valorizes individual flexibility, autonomy, and intrinsic rewards (symbolic capital, creative fulfilment) over stable working conditions, making it a paradigmatic example of neoliberal employment models. Such precariousness within cultural industries contributes to broader sociological debates about exploitation, self-exploitation, inequality, and the erosion of labour rights and protections (Oakley, 2014; Bridgstock, 2011; Comunian & Gilmore, 2016).

In this context, theatre serves as a key illustration of these complexities. Sociologically, theatre represents a crucial intersection of artistic innovation, cultural heritage, community cohesion, and economic sustainability but, as a highly symbolic yet economically fragile sector, theatre highlights the tensions inherent in the cultural and creative industries. Theatrical activities exemplify both the cultural industries' capacity for social engagement and their vulnerability to market pressures, funding constraints, and audience fluctuations (Belfiore & Bennett, 2008; Ferrante & Velani, 2024).

The Theatre Within Cultural and Creative Industries and the Training Needs

Theatre holds a distinct and multifaceted role within cultural and creative industries, serving as an artistic form, cultural heritage, social commentary, economic activity, and a tool for social cohesion and community building.

Artistically, theatre occupies a unique position due to its intrinsic performative nature. Fischer-Lichte's concept of the 'transformative power of performance' (2005) encapsulates theatre's capacity not merely to represent but to enact cultural and social realities actively, thus shaping audience perceptions, attitudes, and social identities. Theatrical performances can create safe and open spaces for confronting and addressing social tensions, cultural differences, and political debates. By enabling diverse voices and marginalized groups to articulate their experiences publicly, theatre contributes significantly to social inclusion and democratic cultural participation.

Additionally, theatre often functions as an incubator and experimental laboratory for creative talent and innovative practices, setting artistic standards and driving broader cultural trends within the creative industries. Emerging theatre artists frequently explore cutting-edge issues, employing experimental methods to develop original dramaturgical languages and innovative theatrical forms. This experimental character of contemporary theatre demands advanced training paradigms and continuous professional development, emphasizing artistic research, creative problem-solving, critical thinking, and interdisciplinary collaborations. Training programmes should, therefore, incorporate pedagogical approaches that nurture experimentation, adaptability, resilience, and the capacity to navigate uncertainty and complexity, reflecting contemporary theatre's dynamic and fluid nature.

Socio-economically, theatre activities stimulate local economies by attracting audiences, fostering related services like hospitality and tourism, and contributing to urban regeneration projects. Policymakers recognize the potential of creative sectors to attract investment, enhance quality of life, and stimulate innovation-led economies, prompting strategic initiatives such as creative city planning, cultural district development, and public–private cultural collaborations. Theatre often acts as a core pillar within these strategies, frequently serving as catalysts for urban regeneration, cultural tourism, and community engagement (Bertacchini & Santagata, 2012).

The presence of vibrant theatrical scenes in cities is closely associated with broader urban renewal efforts, attracting creative talent and enhancing urban spaces' cultural attractiveness (Comunian & Gilmore, 2016). Moreover, theatre significantly impacts employment through direct and indirect channels, supporting professionals in acting, directing, stage management, scenography, costume design, marketing, and technical services. The sector thus generates economic value while simultaneously nurturing creative skills, craftsmanship, and artistic innovation.

Furthermore, contemporary theatre has increasingly integrated digital technologies and innovative multimedia approaches, extending its boundaries and audience-engagement strategies. Digital innovation offers theatre companies novel avenues for creating hybrid experiences, blending traditional theatrical elements with digital storytelling techniques, virtual reality, augmented reality, and interactive platforms (Santagata, 2009). These technological advancements not only enhance artistic creativity but also transform audience participation models, expanding theatre's reach across diverse and globalized communities. The Covid-19 pandemic has dramatically illustrated the fragility and resilience of cultural and creative sectors (Ernst & Young, 2021; Unesco, 2021). The crisis disproportionately impacted theatres, live performances, and cultural venues, exacerbating pre-existing vulnerabilities such as precarious employment and financial insecurity. Yet, the pandemic also accelerated digital innovation within these industries, stimulating creative responses, digital experimentation, and adaptation strategies that might fundamentally alter the future trajectory of creative sectors. Sociological analyses emphasize how these transformations are reshaping the industry's training needs, requiring increased digital fluency, innovative audience-engagement techniques, crisis management capabilities, and hybrid business models integrating digital and physical cultural experiences (Banks, 2020). Theatre practitioners today require training and education encompassing technical proficiency, digital literacy, interdisciplinary collaboration, and adaptive creative skills to thrive within rapidly evolving technological environments.

Nevertheless, even though theatre has an important cultural, social, and economic impact, it faces many sustainability challenges and uncertainties. The financial issues, changing patterns of funding, precarity of employment, and increasing competition for audiences are all pressing issues theatre workers face. Because of this precarity, there must be an education approach that teaches theatre practitioners broad skills including entrepreneurial skills, cultural management skills, audience development skills, and advocacy skills to deal with structural and systemic issues that theatre practitioners face (Scandurra, 2015).

Ultimately, the role of theatre as a custodian of cultural heritage and identity should be acknowledged. Theatre is a cultural archive, sustaining traditions, ritual, narratives, and artistic activity across time. By way of educational programming, public engagement, and community-based work, theatre conserves cultural memory and nurtures intercultural exchange. Theatre functions to connect historical continuity with contemporary innovation, highlighting its potential as an educational tool and the need for training programmes that connect historical knowledge and contemporary artistic and technical knowledge.

In summary, theatre as part of the cultural and creative industries represents compound intersections between artistic creativity, social responsibility, technological innovation, economic activity, and cultural heritage practices and preservation. Training and education strategies in theatre also need to capture these intersections to prepare professionals with broad, robust skill sets to work towards addressing emergent issues and harness theatre's substantial social, economic, and cultural impact.

The Emerging Importance of Soft Skills: The Case Study of Friuli Venezia Giulia

Within Italy, theatre operates under a highly fragmented and decentralized institutional framework. While the major national funding bodies support large theatres or more well-known festivals consistently, smaller or independent theatre companies experience serious financial issues and continue to exist within continuous cycles of short-term funding applications with little long-term stability in programming. This has led to professional operational contexts that include, uncertainty about finances, short-term contracts, irregular income, job precarity, and very limited access to welfare (Belfiore & Bennett, 2008; Scandurra, 2015). These structural conditions have significant influences on different pathways of professional careers, professional development needs, and theatre institutions' capacity to create and sustain long-term strategies and programming. Similarly, several countries across Europe and beyond are increasingly adopting neoliberal cultural policies characterized by reducing direct funding allocations, an increasing emphasis on market-driven strategies, private sponsorship, and the ideals of financial sustainability. Such policy shifts further exacerbate precarity among theatre practitioners, forcing them to develop entrepreneurial capabilities, commercial skills, and innovative managerial competencies previously less emphasized within traditional artistic education (Schonmann, 2015). These transformations in theatre systems underline the urgent necessity of integrating managerial, entrepreneurial, and technological competencies into theatre curricula.

According to Bridgstock (2011), the contemporary creative economy necessitates diverse competencies extending beyond conventional artistic or technical skills. While technical proficiency in specific disciplines—such as design, performance arts, media production, or digital technologies—remains foundational, the modern creative professional must also possess cross-disciplinary abilities, including entrepreneurial acumen, flexibility, innovative thinking, and adaptability to rapidly evolving market demands.

Higher education institutions frequently fail to offer adequate integration between creative practices, entrepreneurial knowledge, and industry-specific competencies required by contemporary creative labour markets. Thus, there exists a significant mismatch between educational outputs and industry expectations, resulting in skill gaps that inhibit workforce readiness, limit employment opportunities, and perpetuate precarious working conditions (Oakley et al., 2008, 2017).

In 2019, the Autonomous Region of Friuli Venezia Giulia promoted a study for the establishment of a 'Technical Professional Pole for Cultural and Creative Sectors'. This initiative, established by national law no. 35/2012, represents an organizational model aimed at facilitating a territorially coordinated education and training offer among technical institutes, professional institutes, and vocational training pathways. It is intended to be aligned with the educational needs arising from production processes and integrated with the economic and productive system.

For several years, the Region has actively supported the cultural and creative sector through the establishment of the 'Culture and Creativity' Cluster. This support aims to enhance visibility and attractiveness, encourage participation in cross-border and transnational European programmes, initiate repositioning and specialization processes of regional enterprises within highly technological production segments, support certified business incubators within the regional territory, issue calls for project initiatives facilitating encounters between the productive sector and creative industries, and organize the first sector-specific fair—Eureka 2022—to foster information exchange and matchmaking between cultural-creative enterprises and traditional businesses. Within the region, the sector has created added value exceeding €2 billion (6% on the regional economy), employing around 33,000 individuals (Symbola, 2024). In 2023, approximately 4000 hires were projected within the sector, including 920 specifically in the performing arts subsector (Unioncamere, 2023). Such regional economic figures demonstrate the broader potential of cultural industries as engines of local economic growth.

The study for the creation of the Technical Professional Pole carried out an in-depth study of the sector's training needs, also involving, through focus groups and targeted interviews, the professionals and managers of performing arts: cultural operators, theatre directors, training designers, artistic directors, audiovisual fund managers and artists. The interviews, which took place in the summer of 2022, focused on two main aspects: the technical and interpersonal skills and abilities required by the sector and difficult to find, and the training tools and supports that are lacking to complement the skills and abilities of young people in the sector (Zago, 2023).

Concerning the first point—skills and abilities required—the sector requires a balanced combination of both technical and relational competencies. Successful professionals in the sector must blend artistic expertise, practical technical know-how, and interpersonal skills.

Within the performing arts, the professionals must possess specific technical skills including technical production skills (lighting techniques, audio engineering, digital editing, broadcasting technology operations), stage and event management (stage setup and operations, safety regulations compliance, ticketing and booking management systems), creative development (screenwriting and script editing, musical composition and orchestration), performance skills (acting, voice modulation, choreography), digital skills (social media management and digital marketing, content creation for streaming platforms, management of online distribution channels).

> In the arts sector, social presence is crucial. Not only for one-way content production but, above all, for community management, conversation management or creative brainstorming.

But this sector places particular emphasis on hands-on manual skills, combined with innovative techniques: artisanal skills (proficiency in traditional craftsmanship methods, high-quality artistic production techniques), design and innovation (product design and prototyping skills, creative use of new materials and technologies), commercialization and business management (e-commerce platform management, branding, marketing, and product positioning skills, understanding of market dynamics and consumer behaviour).

An essential area identified by numerous interviewees as requiring substantial attention within training frameworks is the development of entrepreneurial and business management competencies (Daniel & Daniel, 2015).

> The biggest problem is the availability of cultural managers. It is a problem because projects increasingly require administrative work. To work in this sector, you must have a fixed team that implements projects and follows them through all phases.

Entrepreneurs and freelancers increasingly dominate the creative labour market, necessitating robust entrepreneurial abilities—including financial literacy, strategic planning, market awareness, intellectual property management, and networking capabilities. Moreover, operators underline the importance of entrepreneurial and managerial competencies in navigating the precarious and unpredictable conditions typical of creative work.

Creative industries frequently involve short-term contracts, project-based employment, freelancing, and high levels of self-employment, highlighting the need for training programmes emphasizing self-management, resilience, networking skills, and entrepreneurial attitudes (Oakley, 2014).

> In the cultural sector, I feel the lack of a spirit of entrepreneurship where technical competence is combined with an ability to achieve results, to complete projects within a set timeframe.

> What is needed is to cultivate from primary to secondary school, also involving parents, a path that students must take of self-awareness because in this way they arrive predisposed to listening, to receiving input, even entrepreneurial input, and opportunities where we talk about how to do business.

In addition to managerial and digital skill demands, the operators identify the critical importance of intercultural competence, collaboration, and networking capabilities within contemporary theatre practice. Theatre production increasingly involves international co-productions, collaborative residencies, and cross-cultural exchange projects. Professionals must navigate complex intercultural interactions, requiring education models that foster cultural awareness, linguistic proficiency, and collaborative approaches to artistic production and management. The ability to build extensive professional networks is also essential for securing partnerships, accessing funding opportunities, and achieving greater artistic visibility (Schonmann, 2015).

> Whoever organises events must learn to speak the language of the guests, be close to their knowledge, which means informing, studying and relating in the right ways. But one must also know how to be curious.

This last point brings out a demand that emerged in every interview: technical competences (hard skills) are important but can be learned and still require constant updating; what is more difficult to find are young people who are also trained in soft skills. Creative sectors rely heavily on collaborative and interdisciplinary project-based environments, demanding professionals who can effectively work in dynamic teams, engage diverse audiences, and build strategic partnerships. Stakeholders consistently highlighted these skills as essential.

- Teamwork and collaboration: Because of the joint nature of cultural projects, an understanding of teamwork as a collaborative practice in multidisciplinary teams is critical.
- Problem-solving and adaptability: As professionals encounter barriers as an intrinsic part of their creative processes (many of which will be unpredictable), they must demonstrate resilience, flexibility, and creative thinking capacity to solve problems.
- Autonomy and responsibility: Because there is frequent self-direction or small team working, workers in cultural work sectors must operate with extreme ownership and self-motivate.
- Curiosity and continuous learning: The rapidity of technological change and changes in audience tastes requires professionals to be continually curious and proactive learners.
- Initiative and entrepreneurial spirit: Because many jobs are independent or freelancers (to an extent), economic development and business management jobs require greater and greater entrepreneurial skills (working towards self-employment), strategic thinking, and self-promotion.
- Empathy and interpersonal communication: Professionals in the cultural effort regularly deal with a variety of audiences (individual and community) and their stakeholders/audiences require a considerable amount of emotional intelligence and communication skill.
- Management of stress and emotional intelligence: The high-stakes and intense nature of the creative production cycle (just within the cycle of production experience themselves—which is time limited) and performance pressure require production experience professionals to mindfully manage their stress and emotional intelligence.

Stakeholders highlight the structural factors contributing significantly to recruitment difficulties for the sector. They note insufficient availability of locally trained talent, leading many businesses to recruit from outside the region, increasing costs and logistics difficulties for smaller cultural businesses. Older professionals approaching retirement are not adequately replaced by younger trained professionals, leading to loss of crucial experience, especially in heritage conservation and traditional artisanal crafts. Stakeholders reported difficulty attracting and retaining younger workers due to irregular hours, seasonal employment, project-based contracts, and relatively low remuneration but also because a wrong perception of cultural employment opportunities.

> Our realities must have direct visibility to the end user, but this visibility is also important for future professionals. If a trained young person is not at all familiar with the realities of his area and does not understand the opportunities that could open up, he becomes a wasted resource.

> First, children must be taught that one can make a living with art. Most parents send their child to school to learn a job; culture is an accessory. This is also a point to be insisted on by educational institutions.

Ultimately, the current training and education programmes were criticized for relying on excessively theoretical approaches, being unaligned with industry needs, and ultimately lacking any degree of field-based experience and/or internships, which made graduates poorly prepared for the market. Stakeholders noted that there was a lack of appropriate internships and apprenticeships for too short a period of time or fundamentally did not provide students with the required skills and competencies.

The stakeholders suggested that one way to address these gaps is to increase the number of experiential or hands-on learning opportunities and suggested developing internships or apprenticeships that are longer and more rigorously articulated within industry contexts to better prepare graduates for the working world. Stakeholders also advocated for more a close and continuous working relationship between educational institutions and industry representatives to regularly develop curricula that incorporates ongoing changes to the market that are reflective of practice.

Another important gap identified was the need for straightforward professional development and training opportunities to fill the identified skill gaps, including working with digital technology, specialized audiovisual skills, cultural management, marketing, and event management. Stakeholders strongly endorsed mentorship for supporting smooth transitions from the academy to the industry context, continued skill development, and professional development. Finally, stakeholders proposed investments in educational infrastructure that reflect current professional technologies and practices (digital skills and techno-literacy).

As creative projects demonstrate the often-complex nature of collaboration across disciplines, these professionals must develop behaviours that can sustain the personal relationships, negotiate alternative perspectives, and understand how to build more inclusive work practices. For that reason, training programmes also need to address the integration of soft skills such as collaboration, adaptability, critical thinking, intercultural competency, communication, and social networking.

Finally, stakeholders stressed the value of lifelong learning and continuous professional development within creative industries, given the rapid pace of change and innovation inherent in these sectors. Cultural and creative professionals require regular opportunities for skills upgrading, knowledge updates, and career guidance to remain competitive in increasingly globalized, technologically evolving markets. Institutional and policy-level support for lifelong learning initiatives, professional training centres, workshops, mentorship programmes, and peer networks become essential components in cultivating resilient, adaptable creative careers.

Final Remarks

In closing, addressing training needs in cultural and creative industries, and specifically in the sector of performing arts, involves developing comprehensive, multidisciplinary educational strategies that integrate creative, entrepreneurial, digital, managerial, and interpersonal competencies. Enhancing alignment between educational curricula and industry requirements is not merely a practical concern but represents a significant challenge, deeply intertwined with questions of equity, identity, sustainability, and the future development of creative economies.

Stakeholders expressed clear concern about the mismatch between available educational programmes and industry demands, as well as wider structural barriers (economic, cultural, and bureaucratic) affecting talent attraction and retention. Particularly, they emphasized the need to shift perceptions to attract highly motivated talent to cultural careers because cultural and creative jobs are often viewed as less prestigious, insecure, and low paying compared to other professional sectors. Measures to professionalize and improve the attractiveness of cultural and creatives' careers, such as clear career pathways, mentorship opportunities, improved remuneration, and greater job stability, should be prioritized by national and local policymakers as it is important to implement targeted communication and promotional campaigns to enhance societal recognition of the cultural sector's economic value and professional viability.

Ultimately, bridging today's training gaps is not just about equipping individuals with skills in communication, organization, event or season planning, or other; it is about shaping a resilient, inclusive, and innovative cultural workforce that will define the creative landscape of tomorrow and contributing to preserve our humanity, as theatre itself emerged from storytelling around the fire—one speaking, another listening. Without this essential interaction, we risk becoming isolated individuals: hermits.

References

Adorno, T., & Horkheimer, M. (2002). *Dialectic of enlightenment (original work published 1947)*. Stanford University Press.

Banks, M. (2020). The work of culture and C-19. *European Journal of Cultural Studies, 23*(4), 648–654.

Belfiore, E., & Bennett, O. (2008). *The social impact of the arts: An intellectual history*. Palgrave Macmillan.

Bertacchini, E., & Santagata, W. (2012). *Atmosfera creativa*. il Mulino.

Boccella, N., & Salerno, I. (2017). Industrie culturali ed economia creativa. Il rapporto con lo sviluppo locale ed il capitale sociale. *LaborEst, 15*, 21–25.

Bridgstock, R. (2011). Skills for creative industries graduate success. *Education & Training, 53*(1), 9–26.

Comunian, R., & Gilmore, A. (2016). *Higher education and the creative economy: Beyond the campus*. Routledge.

Daniel, R., & Daniel, L. (2015). Enhancing capacity for success in the creative industries: Undergraduate student reflections on the implementation of work-integrated learning strategies. *Asia-Pacific Journal of Cooperative Education, 16*(3), 199–209.

De Voldere, I. et al. (2017). Mapping the creative value chains. A study on the economy of culture in the digital age. European Commission. https://op.europa.eu/en/home.

Ernst & Young. (2021). *Rebuilding Europe: The cultural and creative economy before and after the Covid-19 crisis*. EYG.

European Commission. (2021). *Updating the 2020 new industrial strategy: Building a stronger single market for Europe's recovery (communication 350 final)*. European Commission.

Ferrante, D., & Velani, F. (2024). *Spettacolo dal vivo: Nuovi autori per nuovi pubblici. Stato dell'arte e prospettive di sistema*. FrancoAngeli.

Fischer-Lichte, E. (2005). *The transformative power of performance: A new aesthetics*. Routledge.

Florida, R. (2002). *The rise of the creative class, and how it's transforming work, leisure, community, and everyday life*. Basic Books.

Florida, R. (2012). *The rise of the creative class, revisited*. Basic Books.

Hesmondhalgh, D. (2019). *The cultural industries* (4th ed.). Sage.

Oakley, K. (2014). Creativity and inequality: The paradox of creative employment. *International Journal of Cultural Policy, 20*(2), 145–161.

Oakley, K., Laurison, D., O'Brien, D., & Friedman, S. (2017). Cultural capital: Arts graduates, spatial inequality, and London's impact. *American Behavioral Scientist, 61*(12), 1510–1531.

Oakley, K., Sperry, B., & Pratt, A. C. (2008). The art of innovation. *International Journal of Cultural Policy, 14*(2), 185–200.

Pignatti, A. (2021). Il settore dello spettacolo nei finanziamenti europei. *Economia della Cultura, 3*, 441–449.

Santagata, W. (2009). *Libro bianco sulla creatività. Per un modello italiano di sviluppo*. Università Bocconi Editore.

Scandurra, G. (2015). Lavorare nel teatro: Note sociologiche su professioni e precariato. *Sociologia del Lavoro, 137*, 37–52.

Schonmann, S. (2015). *International yearbook for research in arts education: Theatre education*. Waxmann Verlag.

Symbola. (2024). *Io sono cultura. L'Italia della qualità e della bellezza sfida la crisi*. Symbola.

Unesco. (2021). Cultural and creative industries in the face of Covid-19: An economic impact outlook. : Unesco.

Unioncamere. (2023). *Imprese e professioni culturali e creative. I fabbisogni professionali e formativi delle imprese culturali e creative*. Unioncamere.

Vilares, M., Rausell, P., & Martínez, C. (Eds.). (2022). Measuring the cultural and creative sectors in the EU. The Measuring CCS Consortium. https://www.measuring-ccs.eu

Zago, M. (2023). I fabbisogni formativi del comparto culturale creativo. In A. Mortara & R. Scramaglia (Eds.), *Cambiamenti in un mondo instabile. Ambiente, tecnologia e consumi* (pp. 151–170). Lumi.

Chapter 8
Their Story, Our History: Some Conclusions After First Post-Lockdown Live Stage Performances: An Experience in Madrid and Sevilla: ON AIR, 2021

Laia Falcón

Introduction

> "fear must be understood not just in terms of the mechanics of selfprotection, but also in terms of the pervasive climate of the times".
> (Scheibe, 2017, *The Drama of Fear,* p. 75)

> "So wrong seemed the World, I face it with rage/while hopeless I whirled like a mouse in a cage, / till you came in range not that life was worth!/ Then presto changed, I'm the happiest girl on Earth!"
> (Cole Porter, 1946, *Look What I Found!*, *Around the World in 80 Days*)

There was a common introduction used by the first scientific publications on medical and social consequences of COVID-19, no matter the specific approach of their authors: when the World Health Organization (WHO) pronounced an official pandemic on March 11th 2020, after 125,000 detected cases in 118 countries (WHO, 2020), the world that we knew changed forever (Cheng et al., 2021; Lara et al., 2021; Mars et al., 2022; Eklund et al., 2022). The epidemic was described as "the greatest stress-causing event worldwide, (…) an unprecedented global challenge (...) also for mental healthcare (…) associated with mental health challenges related to morbidity and mortality caused by the disease and to mitigation activities, including the impact of physical distancing and stay-at-home orders" (Czeisler et al., 2020 in Cheng et al., 2021, 1).

Social isolation operated both as an extremely needed norm to slow the transmission, and as a severe cause of "loneliness, financial burdens, and impairment of individuals' health and well-being" (Brooks et al., 2020, 395). With such a common gigantic enemy, suddenly the world became a community: a "we", totally immersed

L. Falcón (✉)
Universidad Complutense de Madrid, Madrid, Spain
e-mail: lfalcon@ucm.es

P. Corvo, I. Riccioni (eds.), *Theatre and Quality of Life*, Social Indicators Research Series 91, https://doi.org/10.1007/978-3-032-09731-6_8

in one of those rare and tragic historical chapters in which, borrowing Scheibe's words, "fear was overt and manifest". In an overwhelming way, even space and time seemed to turn into collapsing pillars since, all at once, there was no country to run away in order to be safe, and there was not enough time to find certitudes. Worldwide dependence on science's findings was of the most extreme urgency... but such extreme urgency dramatically clashed against science's procedures, which depend on time to get valid solutions.

One year after the declaration of the pandemic (that is, 2021, the year on which this research is focused) collective fear and mourning were still at the basis of the daily life of many, trying to deal with the death of millions, the remaining needs of restrictions and the overwhelming lack of certitudes (Berasategi Santxo et al., 2021). In 2021 population in Spain was still trying to socially react to recent facts of immeasurable impact: just 1 year before, people weren't allowed to visit their beloved ones in cases of imminent death related to COVID-19; and, due to the high number of corpses in some cities, leisure places had to be used as improvised morgues. How does a community talk about such a reality? And how does a social group talk about the need to physically meet again or laugh together again, after such risk of contagion and such intensity of pain? Particularly in collective processes of such complexity the social production of meaning strongly depends on certain key institutions, among which art (and theatre in a very specific and powerful way) plays a significant role (Corbin et al., 2021; Diener & Seligman, 2004; Sandhu et al., 2021; Seligman, 2002; Urke et al., 2021; Riccioni, 2021). Resuming the theories of Aristotle, Nietzsche or Simmel, it is particularly meaningful how Riccioni synthesizes the role of theatre in such process: through "the art of manifesting what is not socially manifest, [theatre] shows the hidden through the mask, (…) becomes a form of 'negative' of society" and therefore helps "to let a society understand the bounds of reason" (Riccioni, 2021, 437).

During the first months after lockdown, the specific nature of theatre experience—based on the co-presence of performer(s) and spectator(s)—turned the act of "going back to theatre" into an intense action of reunion and reciprocal encouragement. The analysis of what happened in live performances during first phases of de-escalation therefore brings an outstanding field for sociological and anthropological research, extremely valuable for the better understanding of collective reinstatement of well-being through art and culture. Aiming to join such lines of research from the analysis of a specific case, this chapter focuses on a theatrical experience developed in Madrid and Sevilla in 2021, when restrictions had still to be notably strong in Spain and collective alert and emotional tiredness were nevertheless significantly intense: the first live performances of the chamber play *ON AIR* (premiered in Madrid's *Auditorio Nacional* in April and in Sevilla's *Espacio Turina* in December), particularly highlighted by spectators, performers, and reviews as an outstanding experience of collective restoration of well-being. Following pages focus on the results of the analysis of open interviews with spectators and performers. However, it may also be relevant to add such shared opinion by mentioning the agreement among reviewers, expressed by both including specific mention of the emotional impact of the show on the audience and specifically describing the performances as a "catharsis" (see Gómez Espinosa, 2021; Pavón, 2021; Reverter, 2021; Thallium, 2021; Vayón, 2021).

In order to consider the collective emotional context of the case and to underline the pertinence of including and comparing both performances, it is important to note that both April and December 2021 were particularly challenging months for Spanish society. April was near the first anniversary of the pandemic, which means also the first anniversary of the highest phase of daily deaths and of the lockdown. After the first year of such collective trauma, the most significant part of society in Spain seemed to face the situation with a combination of mixed feelings: in general terms, there was an obvious will of celebration towards the successful decrease of daily deaths as a collective enormous victory; on the other hand, there was also a strong feeling of alert, sadness, and emotional tiredness because COVID-19 was still causing deaths and strong restrictions were still needed. Unfortunately, in December the pandemic was still far from resolved, and the population in Spain had to deal with reinforced restrictions, including a very low and strict limit of participants in social gatherings (quite a challenging and symbolic norm for many during the Christmas season).

Methodology: Observing and Interviewing About Emotional Impact and Well-being

This research focuses on two main aims. The first one is to explore the dynamics of the emotional impact in terms of a restored sense of collective well-being identified by performers and spectators of these two chosen performances. The second one is to examine the theatrical decisions of adaptation that, according to the historical context, led in this case to such results.

A qualitative study has been applied, based on two key approaches. The first one has been the systematic observation of the process: the adaptation of the piece and the rehearsals. The second one follows the methodology employed by Walmsley in his research on the personal and intrinsic aspects of impact "as articulated by theatre-goers themselves" (Walmsley, 2013, 74), applied in this case to the analysis of 46 semi-structured interviews. Though Walmsley focuses on spectators, he also includes a small sample of professional theatre workers (artistic directors, general managers, and marketing managers) as a comparative insight (Walmsley, 2013, 79, after Bergadaà & Nyeck, 1995). Due to the significant historical context of this case, this research adapted such comparative insight as an opportunity to include the performers. The interviews' length was 30 min each and they were conducted by the same researcher (the 40 spectators' interviews through online or telephonic conversations; the 6 performers' interviews through face-to-face meetings).

Adapting Walmsley's sample of profiles, the category "country of residence" was replaced by "place and date of the performance" and two more categories were added: "country of origin" and the "role" played during the performance. Regarding the performers, three different artistic roles were clear, but in the case of the audience such difference was used to identify those who had decided to attend the performance in 1940's costumes (following the invitation communicated by the advertising of the performances, at the purchase of the tickets, and in previous media interviews and reports). Since the age range of participants (from 6 to 79 years) includes an interesting number of children and childhood was indeed a highly relevant segment of population regarding social resilience and cope (Sancho et al., 2021), school level was added to the category of Education. There are no women among the performer participants because the only female performer taking part in the piece (the singer) is, in fact, the author of this research. The sociodemographic profile of the participants is displayed in Tables 8.1 and 8.2:

Table 8.1 Profile of audience participants

Place and date of the performance	Country of origin	Gender	Age	Education	Role
Madrid, April: 20	Spain: 29	Female: 23	Under 10: 6	School: 6 School leaver: 1 Degree 7 Higher degree: 26	Disguised in 1946's style: 13
Sevilla, December: 20	Andorra:1	Male: 17	10–20: 3		Non-disguised: 27
	Portugal: 1		20–29: 3		
	Italy: 1		30–39: 3		
	UK: 1		40–49: 9		
	Russia: 1		50–59: 8		
	China:1		60–69: 2		
	Egypt: 1		70–79: 6		
	USA:1				
	Bolivia: 3				
Total: 40	Total: 40	Total: 40	Total: 40	Total: 40	Total: 40

Table 8.2 Profile of performer participants

Place and date of the performance	Country of origin	Gender	Age	Education	Role
Only Madrid, April: 1	Spain: 6	Male: 6	20–29:1	Degree 1 Higher degree: 5	Figurant: 1 (only took part in Madrid's performance)
Both Madrid and Sevilla (April and December): 5			40–49: 1		Musicians: 4
			50–59: 4		Narrator: 1
Total: 6	Total: 6	Total: 6	Total: 6	Total: 6	Total: 6

From Walmsley's list of 11 basic interview questions (Walmsley, 2013, 79), five were selected and adapted:

1. How often have you attended theatre since the end of lockdown? (from "How often do you attend theatre per year?")
2. What have been your main memorable moments of the performance and how did they affect you? (from "What was your first memorable experience of theatre and how did it affect you?")
3. What did you hope to get from going to this performance? (from "What do you hope to get from going to the theatre?")
4. What did you do before and after seeing the play? (from "What do you do before and after seeing a play?")
5. What other activities would you equate with the experience you got from this performance? (from "What other activities would you equate with the experience you get from theatre?")

A Strategy Facing Tragedy: Adapting the Scripts and Staging to Social Context as an Urgent Need for Performances During Pandemic

"The reality being represented must be 'adapted' to the context" (Riccioni, 2021, 441): indeed a theatrical rule, that becomes even stronger in historical chapters of massive danger and loss. In the performances here analysed, the powerful impact of such adaptation was significantly highlighted in participants' interviews: "from the very first tones [of the singing] I started to remember all that we have gone through this last year" underlined one spectator (retired male university professor, aged 71, disguised in 1946's style, who attended Madrid's show); "it was all about *that story in the play*, but also about us, about our history", explained another (female high school student, 17, non-disguised, in Sevilla); "it was so relieving in the last monologue about 'our last worldwide episode' [in the plot, referring to the ending of WWII] and the sense that we were all feeling the same (...) I mean the same as the characters, but also I mean we were all feeling the same on both sides of the stage, we performers and spectators were together, talking about the same, thinking about the same" (performer, musician, 53).

Although *ON AIR* was not originally oriented as a specific program for social well-being, it is also clear that its script, musical selection, and main communicative goal aimed to invite spectators to a deep collective reflection about social interaction and multicultural sharing. In the original plan of the project (written 2 years before the pandemic by the same author of this research), the metaphor of the travel drawn by Verne and versioned by Welles was chosen as a key concept to talk about our social need to share and to know "the others" from their own stories: in the first script presented in February 2020 to the head manager of the music festival of

Madrid's Universidad Autónoma, the free adaptation of this play mixed Porter's songs from *Around the World in 80 days* with original songs from other countries of the travel (France, Italy, Egypt, Russia, India, China, Japan...) to be performed in their own native languages and musical timbres and aesthetics. From its first drafts, the play had a strong will to adapt its script and certain songs to each new chance of performance: a sort of statement of an "adapting identity" and "not ethnocentric will", mostly considering eventual adjustments to new geographical destinations and maybe features that could better fit the personality of certain festivals in the future. The main purpose of such decisions was to underline a clear message, almost in a fairy tale style: by leaving his rigid patterns, by reconsidering his self-centred references, and most of all, by knowing new realities *from their own words and voices*, Verne's hero Mr. Fogg wins an outstanding prize…he listens to people for real, he makes friends for the first time and he returns home as a wiser man (in only 80 days!). This was meant to be a happy ending and intercultural collective celebration of the importance of sharing as a social need, so urgent in the Digital Era. The idea was intended to be enthusiastic and colourful, attractive in its musical complexity and richness, and on February 21st, 2020, the prestigious national festival of the Autónoma University of Madrid hired it for its next season and announced it for April 2021. On February 21st, 2020, this really seemed an ideal situation for a chamber musical theatre project like this: more than a year ahead to engage prestigious musicians and narrator, find figurants, costumes, and stage props, and, most of all, to rehearse and stage according to a fine calendar. With a similar coolness and certitude of Mr. Fogg's, the map and the schedule seemed to be perfectly under control: nothing could go wrong. Then, 3 weeks after that, the world changed in the most dramatic way: on March 12th, WHO pronounced the pandemic, on March 13th, Spain entered the national Alarm State; on March 14th, lockdown was decreed for the whole country.

During the first 3 months of lockdown—while the first deaths of friends occurred and that state of collective grief and fear began—the play started an adaptation towards a much more explicit connection between our present and the time of Welles and Porter's play (1 year after WWII). The link between the two historical periods was already pointed out in the first drafts, since many original staging decisions were meant to place the show in a 1946's ambience even before the start of the performance: the playbill's information (the date and the artists' biographies and pictures) were formulated as in 1946; the entrance of audience and performers would be simultaneous and planned to imitate how it would have been in a radio theatre hall in the 1940's; and not only performers would be supposed to wear 1946's costumes, even the audience would be invited to attend the venue in a "1940's flair" ("a hat or a handbag of your grandparents will do", was the line decided to be included in the advertising and ticket selling). Together with such pre-show and stage decisions, during the pandemic some modifications were added in order to intensify the connection between these two historical periods of worldwide loss and grief: the order of the songs was modified to reinforce the link between the climax and the key concept of nearness; more direct references to spectators were added to the dialogues ("don't you think, dear ladies and gentlemen?", "isn't it so, dear audience?") to reinforce their inclusion and their identification with 1946's spectators; comical gags were added as relieving parentheses, in contrast to intense emotional sections; and a new pre-final monologue on "what we all have gone through during recent times" was added, referring in the plot to the tragedy of WWII but very explicitly linked to contemporary pandemic worldwide social fear and loss.

Riccioni's expression of the key role played by "the spectator of the time" (Riccioni, 2021, 441) indeed becomes even more intense in cases like this: by representing the spectators of a show being performed in 1946 (that is, people who had just survived WWII and who still were dealing both with collective grief and with social restoration of hope and well-being), *ON AIR*'s audience celebrated an intense sense of reunion, resistance, and relief. Two statements summarize it in a very significant way: "it really felt like being together again", a spectator explained (female film producer, 42, non-disguised, Madrid); "and that thing about being heroes as our grandparents were... about finding the way again, as they did it...that was really something!", underlined another one (female university professor,65, disguised, Sevilla).

"Talking About Us"

It is significant that, for 75% of spectator-participants, these performances were the first return to theatre after lockdown. This is indeed a fact that helps to better understand one of the three main expectations about the show expressed by spectators: "to feel again the feeling of attending together to a live performance" (female teacher at a high school, 40, non-disguised, Madrid). The other two main expectations were related to the will of watching and listening again to those specific performers, and to the interest in the play itself: all children participants proudly underlined that they knew the story from before and liked it very much; and a significant number of adults expressed their will of watching such an "intriguing version and colourful music program" (male engineer, 48, disguised, Madrid). All performers had already participated in public presentations after lockdown, but, except for the wind player (and the mentioned female singer, who is not included in the interviews), this was the first chance to perform without a mask facing the audience (due to theatrical protocols and after negative COVID-19 tests of all the team), a highly celebrated sign of restored artistic well-being.

Before the first show, three performers were concerned about "the quality" of the connection with spectators, since "the obligatory mask and social distance for audience is crucial these days, but may indeed be a difficult barrier for us to really communicate with them (...) is not easy to see their eyes and we don't get their facial expressions, this makes things quite hard" (performer, musician, 51). But, according to testimonies from spectators and performers, the result was very satisfactory regarding this issue: "when I saw some people disguised and artists started to enter the stage as normal radio workers from the 1940's, waving at us, preparing themselves and waiting the show to start as anybody else in the hall, I felt I was *inside the movie* (...) in a few minutes I forgot I wasn't disguised myself and I forgot I was wearing a mask; I simply stopped thinking about it" (male photographer, 47, non-disguised, Madrid).

Among the main "memorable moments of the performance" highlighted by participants, both performers and spectators mentioned the simultaneous entrance in the hall, as "a true moment of reunion" (performer, narrator, 55), "like meeting a friend again, after a long, long time" (female journalist, 52, disguised, Sevilla). The most mentioned "memorable moments" were linked to two issues: the intense emotion and the sense of well-being aroused by the "permanent surprise of a new song in a new language (...) like in a magic show, we were all the time wondering what was going to be the next surprise" (female economist, 36, disguised, Madrid). Among these most memorable moments, almost every adult participant mentioned a similar list: the beginning of the first singing number, the pre-final monologue, the pre-final Bernstein song *My New Friends*, Porter's *Look what I Found* final number, and a song that somehow connected each to their parents or grandparents' music. The international nature of the program, sung in original languages and aesthetics, acted as a key trigger for emotion and well-being, particularly identified with the sense of travel and worldview, but also with memory and connection with previous generations: "*Suspiros* [*de España*] reminded me so much of my mother, it was impossible not to cry" (female retired lawyer, 71, disguised, Sevilla), "in Egypt everybody knows *In rah Menek Ja Ein*, I felt I was at home with them!" (female language teacher originally from Cairo, 56, non-disguised, Madrid); "Rachmaninov song came as a total surprise, we weren't expect it at all, we had goosebumps all over" (female journalist originally from Moscow, 27, non-disguised, Madrid); "I would have never thought I could listen to that song here, I told my parents afterwards and they knew it by heart" (female student in university, 21, originally from Wuxi, non-disguised, Madrid); "those songs were all day through at my parents' radio when I was a girl, I can't express how happy I felt, I would have raised and dance!" (female retired cultural manager and translator originally form Chicago, 79, non-disguised, Madrid).

It is significant that all adult participants shared common answers to the question "What other activities would you equate with the experience you got from this performance?": travelling, dancing, and going to a party. And it is significant too that nearly 80% of spectator participants had arrived at the show directly from their homes but, after the performance, stood near the venue talking for a while: "we started talking at the exit and we stood there for more than 30 minutes" (male writer, 78, non-disguised, Sevilla); "there was this feeling of arriving home after a good flight, everybody talking to each other while waiting for the suitcases" (photographer, 47, non-disguised, Madrid).

New Meanings (and Some Conclusions)

Indeed, at the time of these two theatrical performances, many psychological and emotional collective consequences of the pandemic were still very intense. And it is interesting that, among those consequences, it was highly significant that the permanence of some "new" (or, at least, more intense) meanings of certain daily words and symbols: expressions and images such as, for instance, "World", "around the World", "time", "counting down", "counting the days", "travelling", "not leaving home", "being together"... that somehow had been socially altered since the beginning of the pandemic. Such a collective process of alteration of meanings has been a key factor for this case. Firstly, it turned out to be crucial for the pertinence of the central metaphor and the specific plot of this play and, therefore, for its emotional impact, both in performers and spectators. Secondly, it became highly decisive for the adaptation of the script, as a needed reaction to the new historical context we were living in. And thirdly, this process of alteration of specific meanings (very subtle in some cases, more intense in others) has also turned out to play a significant role in the structure, the inner direction and the vocabulary of the research itself. Because what the worldwide community has experienced during the pandemic gives a new sense to many key expressions and ideas of the Theory of Theater itself: after what we have observed and experienced during these last 3 years, we *read again* the key literature of the Theory of Theater and notice that some fundamental ideas have a fuller and broader meaning. Indeed, for us, as a worldwide community, theatrical key concepts such as "shared breath" or "the truth behind the mask" (Riccioni, 2021, 437,442) have now a broader and more urgent social meaning.

References

Scientific References

Berasategi Santxo, N., Idoiaga Mondragon, N., Ozamiz-Etxebarria, N., & Dosil-Santamaria, M. (2021). Well-being of adolescents in de-escalation situation: Physical, emotional, social, and academic impact. *Frontiers in Psychology, 12*, 646027.

Bergadaà, M., & Nyeck, S. (1995). "Quel marketing pour les activités artistiques: une analyse qualitative comparéedes motivations des consommateurs et producteurs de théâtre." *Recherche et Applications en Marketing (French Edition), 10*(4), 27–45.

Brooks, S. K., Webster, R. K., Smith, L. E., Woodland, L., Wessely, S., Greenberg, N., et al. (2020). The psychological impact of quarantine and how to reduce it: Rapid review of the evidence. *Lancet, 395*, 912–920.

Cheng, G., Liu, J., Yang, Y., Wang, Y., Xiong, X., & Liu, G. (2021). Stressful events and adolescents' suicidal ideation during the COVID-19 epidemic: A moderated mediation model of depression and parental educational involvement. *Children and Youth Services Review, 127*.

Corbin, J. H., Sanmartino, M., Hennessy, E. A., & Urke, H. B. (2021). Arts and health promotion: Tools and bridges for practice, research, and social transformation.

Czeisler, M. É., Lane, R. I., Petrosky, E., Wiley, J. F., Christensen, A., Njai, R., et al. (2020). Mental health, substance use, and suicidal ideation during the COVID-19 pandemic—United States, June 24–30, 2020. *Morbidity and Mortality Weekly Report, 69*(32), 1049.

Diener, E., & Seligman, M. E. P. (2004). Beyond money: Toward and economy of wellbeing. *Psychologial Science in the Public Interest, 6*, 1–31.

Eklund, R., Bondjers, K., Hensler, I., Bragesjö, M., Johannesson, K. B., Arnberg, F. K., & Sveen, J. (2022). Daily uplifts during the COVID-19 pandemic: What is considered helpful in everyday life? *BMC Public Health, 22*, 1–10.

Lara, R., Fernández-Daza, M., Zabarain-Cogollo, S., Olivencia-Carrión, M. A., Jiménez-Torres, M., Olivencia-Carrión, M. D., et al. (2021). Active coping and anxiety symptoms during the COVID-19 pandemic in Spanish adults. *International Journal of Environmental Research and Public Health, 18*(16), 8240.

Mars, L., Arroyo, R., & Ruiz, T. (2022). Mobility and wellbeing during the covid-19 lockdown. Evidence from Spain. *Transportation Research Part A: Policy and Practice, 161*, 107–129.

Riccioni, I. (2021). Forms of public sphere: Theatre as a collective social builder. *Învățământ, Cercetare, Creație, 7*(1), 437–448.

Sancho, N. B., Mondragon, N. I., Santamaria, M. D., & Munitis, A. E. (2021). The well-being of children in lock-down: Physical, emotional, social and academic impact. *Children and Youth Services Review*, 127.

Sandhu, H., Hirose, N., Yui, K., & Jimba, M. (2021). Community theater for health promotion in Japan. In *Arts and health promotion: Tools and bridges for practice, research, and social transformation* (pp. 103–119).

Scheibe, K. E. (2017). *Deep Drama: Exploring life as theater*. Springer.

Seligman, M. E. P. (2002). *Authentic happiness: Uilizing the new positive psychology to realize your potentianl for lasting fulfillment*. Free Press.

Urke, H. B., Hennessy, E. A., Sanmartino, M., & Corbin, J. H. (2021). Exploring the potential for the arts to promote health and social justice. In *Arts and health promotion: Tools and bridges for practice, research, and social transformation* (pp. 3–15).

Walmsley, B. A. (2013). A big part of my life': A qualitative study of the impact of theatre. *Arts Marketing: An International Journal, 3*(1), 73–87. ISSN 2044-2084.

WHO. (2020). WHO Director-General's opening remarks at the media briefing on COVID-19 – 11 March 2020

Quoted Journalistic and Media References

Gómez Espinosa, J. (2021). "Ser o hacer arte (ON AIR: Tarde de teatro con música)", *RITMO*, April the 22nd.

Pavón, J. P. (2021) "Surtido de bombones teatrales en Sevilla", *El Correo de Andalucía,* December the 9th.

Reverter, A. (2021), "Viaje musical bien ilustrado" *La Razón* and *Beckmesser*, April the 23th.

Thallium, M. (2021). "Laia Falcón, triunfo por aclamación", *Scherzo* April the 22nd,

Vayón, P. (2021). "Viaje a la memoria del siglo XX", *El Diario de Sevilla,* December the 7th.

Chapter 9
Terceira and Its Carnival. Community, Theatre, and Quality of Life

Marxiano Melotti

Introduction

The island of Terceira, in the Azores archipelago, hosts each year a Carnival that, as we shall see, can be regarded as one of the most important popular theatre festivals in Europe and perhaps in the world. This celebration, with its highly distinctive features, is not only an important element of local and European cultural heritage worthy of recognition but also plays a fundamental role in the island's identity and social processes, making a decisive contribution to the quality of life and well-being of its inhabitants.

Around its Carnival (which is part of a more complex system of festivities) the island has built a self-representation that—through the image of "the most festive island" and "the amusement park of the archipelago"—manages to restore centrality to a peripheral condition, transforming a stereotype, which conceals a political (and touristic) colonial gaze, into a heritage specificity of which to be proud (Melotti, 2026).

Terceira's Carnival constitutes a self-reflective and self-governed participatory space in which the community stages itself and, year after year, reflects on the transformations that have occurred and on what lies ahead. It tempers and neutralises anxieties, fears, and tensions linked to internal conflicts and frustrations; it serves as a space and instrument for negotiating identity among the island's various components (in territorial, social, political, cultural, generational, and gender perspectives); it contributes inclusively to the intergenerational transmission of the community's value system; it educates younger generations about the importance of respecting tradition and those components, such as the elderly, who have helped build it; and it fosters reflection on the processes that most affect the community's

M. Melotti (✉)
Niccolò Cusano University, Rome, Italy
e-mail: marxiano.melotti@unicusano.it

P. Corvo, I. Riccioni (eds.), *Theatre and Quality of Life*, Social Indicators Research Series 91, https://doi.org/10.1007/978-3-032-09731-6_9

life and quality of life (such as the impoverishment of the middle class, the peripherality of insular life, migratory flows in and out, new multiculturalism, globalisation, and tourism development).

During the 4 days of Carnival, theatrical performances prepared by different groups circulate across the island's numerous stages, turning the island into one large stage. As one of the texts from the 2025 Carnival puts it, the island becomes a "stage of life" (Martins, 2025).

History and Structure of Terceira's Carnival

Inserted in 2020 into Portugal's National Inventory of Intangible Cultural Heritage (MatrizPCI), Terceira's Carnival has a highly distinctive structure—eminently theatrical in nature—which sets it apart from other Carnivals. From a historical perspective, it is generally considered the result, on the one hand, of a long process of reworking and transforming satirical performance practices traceable to early sixteenth-century Portuguese literature, and, on the other, of the island's role as an international and transatlantic crossroads during the golden centuries of Portuguese colonial expansion (Duarte, 2010). More realistically, the current form of this Carnival—bourgeois in character despite the island's long rural identity—can be traced back to the early decades of the twentieth century or, at most, to the late nineteenth century, when "new" urban and bourgeois Carnivals were also emerging in other European countries.

In Terceira's cultural history, the early twentieth century saw tensions between the urban bourgeoisie of Angra do Heroísmo—the main town—and the island's rural reality, organised into village communities (*freguesias*). These tensions contrasted a rural "brutal" street Carnival with a bourgeois "civilised" one, organised inside theatres and private halls (Enes, 1989).

There was certainly a process of mutual hybridisation, evident both in the theatrical dimension and in the importance of musical accompaniment, which even today—despite many innovations—retains a band-like character, rooted not only in the street activities but also in the "philharmonic" culture of music halls widespread across the island. A particular aspect of this Carnival is the high level of musical literacy it presupposes, with dozens of people capable of playing one or more musical instruments at a professional level.

Probably in the 1970s, the various practices merged into the today's form of the Carnival: highly formalised yet very dynamic and varied performances, generally staged indoors on one of the many stages in halls scattered across the island, each representing a different *freguesia*.

There are several types of performance: the *dança de espada* (considered the most noble and sophisticated form, with a dramatic content often moralistic and sometimes religious); the *dança de pandeiro* (in which the musical part is led by a tambourine player who can reach true musical and choreographic virtuosity with the instrument); and the *bailinho* (Falcão Mendes, 2018). These performances, with a formalised structure, involve numerous musicians who, in addition to playing, sing and perform choreographed movements, and actors who recite a text developing a story. Among the narrative sections, the opening *saudação* (greeting) and closing *despedida* are particularly important and serve an identity function: the *mestre* (the musician who leads the orchestra), singing and accompanied by the orchestra—which also acts as a chorus—introduces the performance, thanks the audience and the host *freguesia*, recalls the group's *freguesia* of origin, celebrates the island and its Carnival, usually stressing the importance of traditions and the uniqueness of Terceira.

In addition to these forms, there may be monologues and *comédias* with a small cast of actors.

What is particularly striking about this Carnival is the sheer number of performances prepared and circulated among the island's various stages over its 4 days, and the extent of popular participation—both as protagonists (playing, singing, dancing, acting, and contributing in various ways to the writing and staging of the performances) and as audiences (filling the theatres, often moving from one *freguesia* to another, from theatre to theatre).

Some data give a clearer sense of the phenomenon. The island is divided into 30 *freguesias*, with a number of stages varying from year to year, but usually around 35. Almost all *freguesias* have at least one group preparing a performance (some have more than one group, thus producing and circulating multiple shows). Groups preparing *danças* and *bailinhos* generally comprise 20–30 people, sometimes up to 40. Each group, during Carnival's 4 days, seeks to perform in as many theatres as possible, often repeating the show more than 30 times.

In the 2015 edition, as part of the preparation of the dossier that led to the Carnival's inclusion in the national intangible heritage list, it was calculated that there were 1140 performances involving 59 groups and a total of 1250 people on stage (Falcão Mendes, 2018). In 2025, 71 performances were staged: 43 *bailinhos*; 12 "senior" *bailinhos* produced by retirement homes, social centres, and seniors' groups; 2 *bailinhos*—one of them "senior"—prepared by Azorean communities in the USA; 7 *danças de pandeiro*; 2 *danças de espada*; 4 comedies; and 1 monologue.

It should be borne in mind that the island has about 56,000 inhabitants. To the number of people involved in producing the shows, one must add the audiences: thousands of people (including children and the elderly) who, for 4 days, from mid-afternoon until late at night, fill the island's various stages. In an inclusive approach, some performances are also taken to nursing homes and senior centres. Some schools prepare their own performances, which are then circulated around the island.

Bretão (1998, p. 19) rightly insists on the popular aspect of this Carnival, an expression of "popular theatre": *do Povo e para o Povo* ("of the people and for the people") of the island. Equally correctly, he recognises the power of these representations, with their mostly simple, direct, and unsophisticated language ("a mental, formal, and verbal production easily received and understood by the popular strata"). In today's cultural context of increasing deintellectualisation of society (Melotti, 2025), this theatrical language proves to be very effective, helping people reflect on the complexity of our world and deal with it.

Research Methodology and State of the Art

This article is the result of a research project launched in 2020 with an international team that also includes faculty from the University of the Azores. During the 2023 and 2025 Carnivals, the author carried out fieldwork involving participant observation, data and material collection, attendance at performances and rehearsals, and, finally, open qualitative interviews with various local stakeholders (public administrators, university professors, local experts, people working in the tourism sector, individuals involved in the preparation and performance of Carnival shows, and residents).

A first outcome of this research was the collective article (Marcelli et al., 2022) devoted to what we defined as the "unknown Carnival" of Terceira: an analysis intended to relate this celebration to the concept of sustainability, based on the premise that culture can be considered one of the pillars of sustainability (Hawkes, 2001) and cultural sustainability is tied to the autonomous development of identities capable of resisting the growing uniformity of models of thought and action (Soini & Birkeland, 2014). Carnival—especially in the active, participatory form it takes in Terceira—is a tool for political and social participation and of collective identity construction through bottom-up dynamics. This approach differs markedly from that of many other contemporary Carnivals, which often rest on top-down processes in which institutions (perhaps even for the benefit of the community itself and with the involvement of some stakeholders) exploit the celebration as a tool for economic development and territorial and tourism marketing, but in doing so limit its most creative and participatory aspects.

Terceira's Carnival, by contrast, manages to exploit and renew a series of traditional Carnival elements (such as the distribution of power and reaction to hegemony), which, along with a mythopoetic process of reinvention and rewriting of local history and strong community participation, contribute to community cohesion (Marcelli et al., 2022).

The research therefore examined the relationship between Carnival and community from an "eco-pedagogical" perspective (Marcelli, 2023), viewing it as a "heritage device" consciously employed by the community as an instrument of informal education to reaffirm annually its relationship with the environment, within the delicate balances of the island space, and to transmit a system of values, including environmental ones, to new generations. Young people and children are systematically involved in Carnival both as spectators in the halls where performances are staged and as members of the groups acting on stage (Fig. 9.1).

From this perspective, we also examined formal education practices—that is, the use of Carnival by the island's schools within a dual heritage and curricular logic. Theatrical performance, prepared at school but included in the "official" performance circuit of the island's Carnival, becomes a tool for heritage education and for the intergenerational transmission of the celebration, which constitutes an important aspect of the island's intangible cultural heritage and, as such, contains the system of values and practices that characterise it.

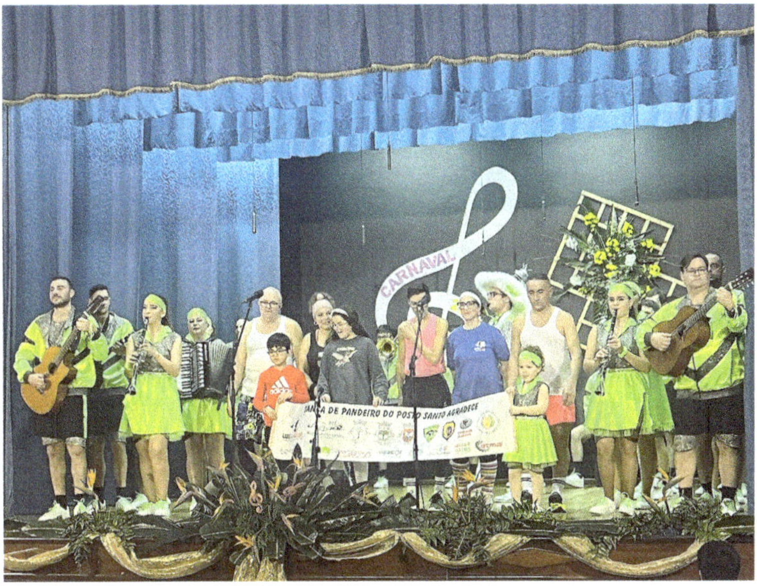

Fig. 9.1 The community on stage. *Dança do Pandeiro do Posto Santo* (2025). Photo of the author

Here theatre reveals its nature as a social practice and, as Paltrinieri (2022) reminds us, as a "performative form of citizenship", of which it is an integral part and fundamental tool, actively contributing to the process of building the social imagination of a community. Moreover, owing to the specific theatrical dimension of this Carnival, the performative activity contributes to acquiring skills in literary and musical education, as well as in study and socialisation (through memorisation of texts, music, and choreography; acting; singing; playing musical instruments; and dancing). This education, in turn, together with intra-family education, enables young people to "enter into" Carnival, to understand its dynamics, and thus to become adults who will help perpetuate the tradition. All these elements, in effect, make the school preparation work for the *dança* a practice of progressive education and active citizenship (Fonseca, 2025).

The Carnival was also examined from a spatialist perspective, focusing on its significance in centre–periphery and local–global dynamics (Melotti, 2026). The subjects, texts, and stage designs of the performances prepared for Carnival depict the dynamic relationship—sometimes conflictual, more often paradoxical—between rural and urban, as well as between local and global. The island, in fact, while still having an economy strongly based on agriculture and livestock, is aware of and participates in global dynamics. This tension between worlds reflects a more complex transformation of the Azorean economy and society (in which, for example, tourism is increasingly important) and constitutes a recurring and evident element within Carnival. Its peculiar theatrical dimension, which includes texts and dialogues, allows it to become a self-reflective space for continuous identity negotiation.

The Political Meaning of This Carnival

In other words, this Carnival presents (and reconfirms every year) a strong "political" meaning, in the sense that it expresses the polis, understood as the community of the island. This aspect in other Carnivals has weakened or been lost in favour of other meanings, perhaps important for the community (such as entertainment, consumption, and tourism) but falling within the broader dynamics of the so-called "carnivalisation of society" (Langman, 2008; Melotti, 2010 and 2019), the process that contributes to depriving Carnival of its uniqueness, weakening its character of rupture, subversion, and suspension (Bachtin, 1941; Caro Baroja, 1979; Fabre 1992).

A comparison with the theatrical festivals of ancient Athens would certainly be bold and misleading, if only for the difference in the quality of the texts (Greek tragedies and comedies not only possess a very high poetic and literary quality, but are also known for having addressed fundamental themes that still structure our way of thinking today). Likewise, it would be simplistic to compare the humour of Carnival texts with the comic structures of Aristophanic theatre, even if some carnival elements can be found in them (Olson, 2025).

However, it is stimulating to reflect on the shared communal and ritual dimension of the performances, as well as on the shared territorial organisation that unites urban and rural (the *polis* is not made up solely of the monumental city but is also expressed in its *chora*). In both cases, theatre—with the necessary differences—constitutes a self-reflective practice for constructing collective identity and citizenship.

Terceira's Carnival, in its specific theatrical and participatory dimension, which includes and represents all the island's *freguesias*, manages to maintain a dense connection with the community. It becomes the community's voice, which from year to year "builds" tradition; reaffirms the importance of the relationship with the past; reflects on the role and image of the island (Fig. 9.2); and highlights and interprets, neutralising them, the fears and anxieties of the present.

The celebration annually (re)builds the community, (re)asserting the presence of each of the realities that compose it (the various *freguesias*, the different age groups, the different social classes—as they would once have been called—and the different family and individual paths), ensuring forms of socialisation that counteract the spatial fragmentation of the island, the (relative) isolation of the island itself, and, more broadly, that recurrent individualist fragmentation of the postmodern condition.

The main difference is that in Terceira, Carnival continues to constitute a central element—living, awaited all year round, not artificial, and above all non-touristic—in the collective imagination and in the social and political practices of the island's various communities. It is not, in short, an "event" constructed for tourist or territorial marketing purposes and is, for now, unaffected by the forms of "eventisation" found in other Carnivals (Melotti, 2026). Nor is it a recently reactivated phenomenon or one reconstructed with a nostalgic, neo-rural, or primitivist logic, as has occurred in several "anthropological" Carnivals of southern Italy (Melotti, 2026).

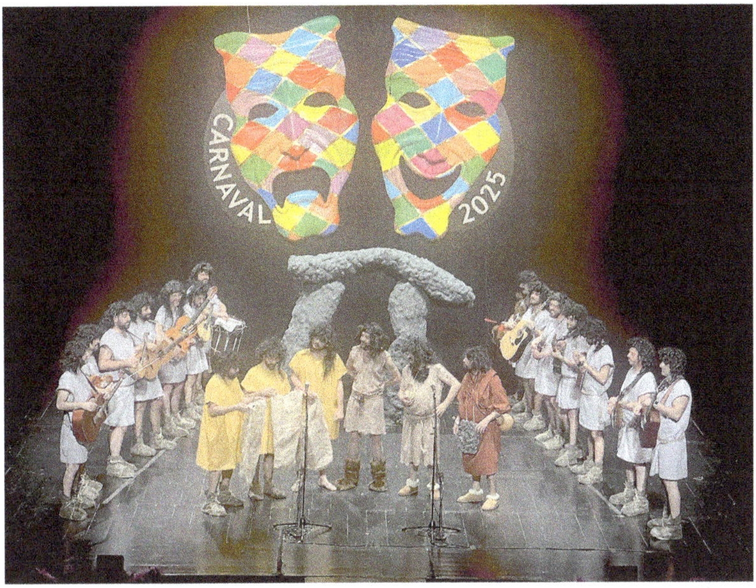

Fig. 9.2 Stonehenge in Terceira. *Grupo Ti-Notas Casa do Povo dos Altares* (2025). Photo of the author

However, we can observe an incipient process of heritagisation, which could, over time, lead to a re-signification of the festival or even to its decline. In 2020, on the initiative of local stakeholders, Terceira's Carnival was included by the Portuguese government in the national inventory of intangible heritage (MatrizPCI, 2016). For now, this inclusion mainly expresses the local community's pride in its cultural history and is part of a legitimate use of intangible heritage by the local community as a positioning tool both in the inter-island dynamics of the archipelago (especially in relation to the main island, São Miguel) and in its relationship with mainland Portugal and the political choices of the central government.

Carnival and the Challenge of Heritagisation

In 2019 Portugal succeeded in obtaining UNESCO recognition as Intangible Cultural Heritage of Humanity for the Carnival of Podence, in the mainland region of Trás-os-Montes. This Carnival is very different from Terceira's and has a more traditional character, closer to the nostalgic tourist gaze that usually accompanies non-urban Carnivals. Official tourist sites, in fact, insist on presenting its masks as "mysterious characters" (Visit Portugal, n.d.), which, on the Municipality's Facebook page (2018), even become "diabolical".

This choice follows the international trend of heritagisation, which, in the name of protecting and enhancing expressions of intangible heritage that might be lost—not to mention the international competition through the number of UNESCO sites and tourism flows—paradoxically risks crystallising and touristifying the heritage it aims to protect (Marcelli et al., 2022). From this perspective, a significant passage from the official website of this festival illustrates the effects of heritagisation and the ambiguous relationship between tradition and what, using a key concept from the sociology of tourism, constitutes a form of "staged authenticity" (MacCannell, 1973): "We are preparing one of the most traditional and authentic events of Portugal! The Entrudo Chocalheiro returns in 2026 with all the strength of its ancestral traditions" (Caretos, 2025).

UNESCO recognition of the "competing" Carnival of Podence has prompted Terceira's administration—for reasons of local pride and also identity and political positioning with respect to mainland Portugal—to seek the same recognition for its own Carnival. The island's municipalities, together with local stakeholders and scholars of the festival, have thus begun preparing a nomination dossier to be presented to the government and to UNESCO. In my view, this is not a secondary aspect, as it can affect the overall meaning of the celebration and therefore its relationship with the community and its well-being.

In the meetings and interviews I had on the island in 2023 and 2025, as regards the UNESCO dossier I never perceived in my interlocutors an intent to heritagise the Carnival for economic or tourist purposes. Of course, some of them were sceptical or concerned about the effects of potential UNESCO recognition. Anyhow, what clearly predominated was pride in the international recognition of the importance of their cultural heritage, accompanied by the belief that their Carnival is so deeply rooted in local culture as not to be at risk of touristification or commodification.

This position, however, tends to underestimate the strength and speed of touristification processes (and more particularly those concerning cultural heritage) and the effect they can exert on the island, on the celebration, on its meaning for the community, and, more broadly, on its well-being and quality of life. Certainly, tourism can contribute to individual well-being and fulfilment (Corvo, 2007) and, as a powerful social factor, can help activate positive practices in the territory (Corbisiero & Monaco, 2025). However, if unregulated, in fragile contexts it ends up eroding the social and cultural fabric of the communities involved, compromising their well-being and altering and trivialising their relationship with their history and their past (Melotti, 2025).

There are, of course, various considerations suggesting that potential recognition is unlikely to have significant repercussions in terms of tourism flows. We know, in fact, that the UNESCO brand can increase tourism (which is why it is sought after by many local communities), but now we also know that—partly because of the ever-growing number of sites and practices recognised by UNESCO as World Heritage—it does not necessarily lead to tourism growth, especially when not accompanied by effective territorial governance practices (Cellini, 2011; Huang et al., 2012; Cuccia et al., 2016).

Moreover, the island's capital, Angra do Heroísmo, has been on World Heritage List since 1983, but this has not entailed an excessive touristification even in high season. This is in contrast to what is happening on the archipelago's main island,

São Miguel, where the continuous implementation of sustainable tourism (see IPDT, 2020)—mainly environmental, sporting, and experiential in nature—is beginning to slide into overtourism, causing great discontent in the local community (Lusa, 2025).

Furthermore, Terceira's Carnival does not correspond to the main types of "tourist gaze" (and thus of tourist stereotypes) usually linked to Carnival. It is not rural, neo-rural, or nostalgic (like Podence, with its "mysterious and diabolical masks"); it is not urban and linked to a playful imaginary (like Viareggio, with its floats bearing imposing papier-mâché figures), romantic (like Venice, with its masked balls, citywide celebrations, and eighteenth-century theming), or sexual (like Rio de Janeiro, with its grand floats and scantily clad dancing women). Moreover, it takes place at a time of year with a climate that is not particularly favourable or attractive.

Above all, however, it is a theatrical Carnival, staged mostly indoors, in theatres, and based on dialogues and songs in the Portuguese language, which, for the most part, refer to themes and figures from local news, often difficult to understand outside the island. Peripherality and self-referentiality thus protect the Carnival from possible tourist-driven decline and from its crystallisation.

Heritage policies, however, can have unwanted effects and attract investors—not necessarily local—interested in promoting tourism development, perhaps of a real estate nature, starting precisely from Carnival (and other island festivities). It should be noted that the Azores Tourism Master Plan, with regard to Terceira, identifies Carnival as a "primary attraction" (IPDT, 2020). It is therefore not unthinkable that the festival could be de-seasonalised and de-contextualised, with performances repeated in the summer or even prepared, perhaps in English, specifically for tourists. This is a practice that is transforming various Carnivals, including "traditional" ones, which, precisely in the name of enhancing their identity and heritage significance, end up being denatured and serialised.

In any case, it is a complex issue, also because the transformation of Carnivals into "events" and their inclusion in post-ritual and territorial marketing dynamics should not necessarily be interpreted as a decline, but can also represent an evolution and adaptation of tradition to the needs of contemporary communities.

What surprised me, however, is that, in the debate surrounding the heritagisation of the local Carnival, the community is so confident in the strength and uniqueness of its Carnival that it does not see tourism as a potentially transformative element—one capable, above all, of altering the relationship between the festival and the community.

The Island Between Isolation and Migration

Terceira is one of the nine islands of the Azores, which constitute an autonomous region of Portugal and are classified among the Outermost Regions of the European Union. The archipelago lies in the heart of the Atlantic: about 1300 km from mainland Portugal, 2300 km from Canada, and 3300 km from the United States. During the age of oceanic exploration and Portuguese colonial expansion, the Azores—and in particular Angra do Heroísmo—played an important role as an Atlantic port of call on the trade routes linking Europe, Africa, America, and Asia. In Angra, a statue dedicated to the great explorer Vasco da Gama still commemorates this glorious past.

This, however, did not prevent substantial flows of Azoreans to the new lands, especially to Brazil, even in the centuries of Portugal's expansion. The gradual loss of Portugal's centrality and the country's lack of industrialisation had significant repercussions on the quality of life in the Azores. Over the course of the twentieth century, there was considerable emigration from these islands to North America, where an important Azorean community took shape (Baganha, 1990; Almeida, 2008). It is only in recent decades that a phenomenon of return migration has been observed (Rocha et al., 2011).

The Azorean diaspora is a phenomenon that has marked—and continues to mark—the culture and identity of the archipelago. On the one hand, it underscores its fragility, tied to a past of poverty and to processes of depopulation and weakening of human capital. On the other, especially in recent decades, it is the basis of a vibrant cosmopolitan identity, with family and community ties, flows of people, material goods, narratives, and experiences connecting both sides of the ocean. This means relationships between very different cultural systems, such as the insular and peripheral context of the Azores—an expression, in any case, of Portuguese culture—and those of areas as varied as mainland Portugal itself, Brazil, Argentina, Canada, and the United States.

The diaspora, in short, has created a network of relationships which, in the case of Terceira, impacts not only the economy (through tourism by emigrants and their descendants) but also the culture and, for our purposes, the festival system. Azorean communities abroad tend to maintain the festive traditions of their places of origin (Leal, 2017; Cordeiro & Formato, 2024) and, as far as Terceira is concerned, prepare Carnival shows (*danças* and *bailinhos*) as on that island.

Every year, for Carnival, one or two groups—sometimes more—arrive on the island to bring to its stages the shows they have prepared. The arrival at the airport of migrants ready to present their performance is always a small event, one that the local press never fails to report. These performances (as often happens with the heritage expressions of diaspora communities) tend to be more traditional than those prepared on the island itself. In the latter, in fact, especially younger participants experiment year after year new languages—with more sophisticated and less band-like musical accompaniments or with a reworking of narrative and choreographic structures. But this is precisely a sign of the vitality of the celebration, capable of building and perpetuating tradition precisely through evolution and constant adaptation to the transformations and differences of the communities that bring it to life.

The island's audiences eagerly await the performances of migrant groups, whose texts display enormous affection for the island and its traditions, but often raise some doubts precisely because of their excessive traditionalism, as I was able to grasp in my interviews.

On the other hand, they follow with interest the innovations of younger authors or musicians—enthusiastically applauded by friends and peers—but express some reservations about excessively innovative sound. But it is precisely this vibrancy and contradiction that makes Carnival a living spectacle, embedded in the socio-cultural fabric of the community.

It should be said that the Terceiran public follows Carnival with a type of engagement that is partly like that of football fans (eagerly awaiting the performance of their own *freguesia* and cheering it on) and partly that of music connoisseurs (judging and commenting on every aspect of the performances, from the plot to the interpretation, as well as the various innovations).

This attitude, in terms of attention, competence, and participation, recalls that of Italian audiences towards opera—especially in past decades and in certain areas more deeply linked to operatic tradition and less transformed by the touristification of opera, increasingly used as a tool for territorial and tourism marketing. (Not by chance, the Italian government—with that same ambiguous attitude between protection and commodification noted above—has sought to have it included in UNESCO's WHL).

Between Centrality and Peripherality: Theatre and the Spatial Dynamics of the Festival

The island, of volcanic origin, is roughly circular in shape. In the central area lies a large caldera, with some fumaroles and three nature reserves. The island's physical structure has meant that settlements have developed essentially along the coast or in inland areas not far from it. The road network is extremely limited: a few roads cut across the island; a short motorway links the airport of Lajes with the two main towns (Angra do Heroísmo and Praia da Vitória). The most important road, however, is the historic one, is the historic one, which runs along the entire coast of the island, crossing and interconnecting the various villages (*freguesias*).

This spatial organisation significantly shapes the daily lives of inhabitants, helping to create a complex urban ecosystem of relationships between environment and settlements, which is also reflected in the island's Carnival and festive system (Melotti, 2026).

From a spatial reading of inter-island relations, the island has no true centre, in the sense that the centre (the caldera) is a non-place, and almost all settlements are located along the coast, in a sort of long and discontinuous circular periphery. Along this coastal line, however, unequal relationships are defined insofar as the succession of rural communities—the *freguesias*—is interrupted by the two aforementioned municipal capitals (one of which in the past was even the capital of the entire archipelago) and by the airport, which, in the logic of today's society of flows, acquires central significance as a place that, symbolically and experientially, interconnects the island with external "centralities" (the island of São Miguel, the capital Lisbon, and, thanks to a direct flight, Boston).

The circularity of the road network, however, tends to assign equal weight to all the settlements along its route (or along the slightly more inland parallel road): all—the towns included—are in the same condition of peripherality with respect to a centre that, in fact, does not exist. Peripherality in relation to the two main towns does not seem to be perceived, insofar as the culture and pride of each *freguesia*—expressed through Carnival—are so strong as to eclipse the predominant administrative role of the two municipal capitals, which, in the performative logic of Carnival, are simply two communities that, like the others, prepare their performances of their *freguesias*.

Terceira's Carnival still shows some traditional elements that many other Carnivals have lost or diluted in the carnivalisation of society. Among them, the increasing complexity of territorial governance forms, the increasingly elusive relationship between social classes and power, the temporary overturning of the established order, and the critique of power. The egalitarianism that characterises it tends to cancel any differences between *freguesias*, as well as between *freguesias* and municipalities. Peripherality and subordination are, therefore, annulled.

The spatial organisation of the festival—based on the circulation of the shows, with an almost circular mobility, shaped by the structure of the island and its road network—contributes to creating a political space that, at the same time, is carnivalesquely utopian and reflects the existing solidarity between the villages of the island. Actually, Terceira's Carnival, by constructing and imposing a performative mobility during its days, helps to nullify any tensions between individuals, groups, and villages.

It is worth noting here that the public can take part in the festival in two ways. They can stay in their own *freguesia* and attend in its theatres (or in one of them) all the shows that arrive in their village or they can move between the various *freguesias* to see specific performances, follow certain groups or construct their own Carnival, with carnivalesque freedom or scientific punctiliousness. As regards mobility, one of the interviewees stated, "I have never seen in mainland Carnivals people moving around so much" (interview in Marcelli, 2023, p. 271).

This intra-island mobility is, of course, part of normal, everyday life (at least since the ease of transport and the spread of cars has made it possible). In the specific festive context, however, it is ritualised, in the sense that it becomes an expected and defining element. As a ritualised component of what is perhaps the island's most important participatory experience, it also becomes a value model, quite different from ordinary daily mobility. In short, the festival teaches circularity and invites the population (in movement from village to village, within each theatre, and within each of the groups) to mingle.

Identity Mythopoeia, Theatre, and New Fears

In the central area lies a large caldera, with some fumaroles and three nature reserves. The terrain, higher in the central zones, slopes down towards the coast: large areas are devoted to agriculture and, above all, to the breeding of cows and bulls.

The latter, in particular, are a distinctive element of the island's economy and history. Their breeding has become a marker of identity and heritage, around which narratives and an actual historical mythopoesis have been built. It is said that a herd of bulls, pushed against an invading army, forced it back into the sea, ensuring the island's independence. This episode is taken as proof of the indomitable spirit of its inhabitants, of whom Brianda Pereira—the heroine who is said to have defended her family and her land in this way—is a model.

In this story we can also detect a nostalgic note for a warlike and glorious past, in which the island played a prominent role: its capital, Angra, was the first settlement in the Azores to be granted the title of "city" in 1534. In 1580, for a few years, Angra was also the capital of Portugal itself and the seat of the royal court, while Terceira was the last Portuguese territory not occupied by the Spanish. Owing to its strategic position as an Atlantic port of call on the trade routes between Europe, Africa, America, and Asia, Terceira played a key role in Portugal's colonial expansion. A statue of the explorer Vasco da Gama stands on Angra's seafront, as a reminder of this past greatness, also attested by buildings that led to the city's inclusion on the UNESCO World Heritage List.

In the early decades of the nineteenth century, Terceira played a role in the Portuguese Civil War, contributing to the liberals' victory over the absolutists. In recognition, the town of Praia was renamed Praia da Vitória, and Angra, again the capital for a brief period, became Angra do Heroísmo. These heroic and warlike events are aspects that its inhabitants of the island like to emphasise, in contrast with the present centrality of São Miguel, the main island of the archipelago.

These mythopoeic elements form the backbone of Terceiran identity and, at the same time, reveal its fragility, in a perpetual oscillation between past and present and between centrality and peripherality. Carnival manages to become a mirror of these and other latent tensions, offering, in a joyful key, reflections that grasp the paradoxical elements of certain processes and help the community overcome them.

It is, in fact, a fundamental tool in the multi-level definition of identity and political relationships: it intervenes in intra-island dynamics (among the different communities of the island); inter-island dynamics (between the various islands of the archipelago, particularly in relations with its main island); between the island and the mainland (and especially with the capital, Lisbon); and, finally, between the island and the rest of the world.

The strength of this Carnival lies precisely in its ability to unite tradition and contemporaneity, absorbing and metabolising a whole series of elements and "signs" of contemporary and postmodern society (the Internet, YouTube, influencers, e-commerce, international pop music, blockbuster films, smartphones, supermarkets, ATMs, tourist resorts, and cruise ships), which are used to demonstrate the island's full inclusion both in competitive dynamics with the other islands and the capital, and in the global dynamics of the consumer and flow society (Melotti, 2026). All of this is related to local dynamics, histories, and issues (difficulty accessing hospitals, population ageing, the persistence of a rural culture, the system of local festivities). Carnival manages to incorporate those global processes that Terceira's inhabitants regard with concern—either because they fear exclusion due to their peripherality or because they are aware of participating in them.

Thus, the island's airport, a constant source of discontent for the delays of its flights, is imagined as being concessioned to an airline from Qatar (*Dança de Pandeiro de São Bartolomeu*). The magical powers of the Genie of the Lamp transform Terceira into a sort of Las Vegas (*Dança de Pandeiro* of the MuTe Project—Escola Básica Integrada dos Biscoitos). An elderly lady, from the rural and "primitive" world of Terceira, finds herself catapulted into the capital, where she is mistaken for a singer and taken to a recording studio (*Dança de Pandeiro António Ivo*). An old woman struggles to use an ATM, and bumbling thieves, after a bank heist, end up enjoying their loot on a tropical beach, assuming the traits of the most stereotypical tourist (*Bailinho das Irmãs Hospitaleiras de A.H.*). Two awkward neighbours become influencers selling bras online (*Dança de Pandeiro das Mulheres de Santa Bárbara*).

As one title proclaims, it turns out that "ABBA were born in Terceira" (*Bailinho dos Rapazes de São Mateus e da Terra-Chã*), and Elvis Presley, alive again, works as a waiter on the island (*Bailinho dos Rapazes de Santa Bárbara*) (Fig. 9.3).

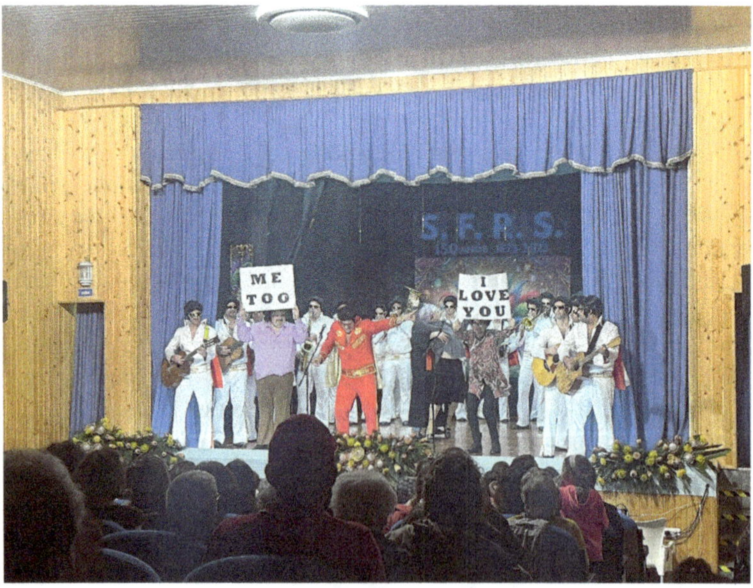

Fig. 9.3 Elvis reborn. *Bailinho dos Rapazes de Santa Bárbara* (2025). Photo of the author

Particularly significant is the script of a *dança de pandeiro* from 2023, prepared by the school of Biscoitos as part of the project mentioned above. In it, cows and bulls (played by costumed children) go on strike, demanding better living conditions that humorously reflect the tourist imagery of contemporary welfare society. The livestock farm goes into crisis. A referendum—including audience participation—resolves the matter, and the bulls return to work. This is not, in short, the ecological and animal rights storyline one might expect from a school, but rather a text teaching children to respect the island's traditions, based precisely on the heroism of Brianda, bull breeding, and *touradas à corda*.

Also noteworthy is a 2025 performance imagining the arrival, 4000 years ago, of a strange tribe of "Neolithic" men in Terceira (Fig. 9.2). These "must progress" and, to meet the expectations of today's scholars and pseudo-archaeologists, decide to build a "megalithic civilisation" in the style of Stonehenge, serving, according to collective imagination, as an astronomical clock (*Ti-notas Casa do Povo dos Altares*).

These very different stories have in common their reflection on, and irony towards, the relationship between peripherality and centrality, and between past and present.

A Pervasive Performance

I am aware that the discussion may seem complex for those unfamiliar with the meaning of *freguesia*: these are small village-level administrative units, originally defined by the presence of a parish. The *freguesias* of Terceira fall under the jurisdiction of two municipalities, which themselves contain *freguesias*. The relationship with the village church remains a significant aspect of daily life and of the *freguesia*'s heritage identity.

This is evident, for example, in the complex festive system of the *Festa do Espírito Santo* (Leal, 1994), where each *freguesia*, in the 8 weeks following Easter, selects (usually on a weekly basis) one or more *Imperadores* who organise and perform the celebrations, creating and renewing a ritual and political space that is distinct both from that of the State and from that of the Church.

The *freguesias* play an important role in the life of the island and are fundamental in building the community cohesion—also expressed through Carnival—that underpins residents' quality of life and well-being. The areas of intervention and activities carried out by a *freguesia*, based on the volunteer work of its members, can be very diverse.

As one inhabitant of Doze Ribeiras recalls, in recent decades the village community has worked together on a series of activities that have significantly improved residents' quality of life: from rebuilding houses heavily damaged by the 1980 earthquake, to widening transit roads in farming areas, to building new drinking-water fountains (interview in Marcelli, 2023, pp. 306–311).

Similarly, it has engaged in activities more directly related to leisure and recreation, such as sport (organising a football team and building a training pitch) or setting up picnic areas and seaside facilities. In Doze Ribeiras, the *freguesia*, at the initiative of its members, also created a cultural association to promote the village's folkloric traditions.

It is within the *freguesia* that the groups animating Carnival take shape, preparing the *danças* or *bailinhos* that will be performed on the *freguesia*'s stage and then toured around the island—a demanding task that begins many weeks (often months) before Carnival and involves groups of 20–30 people (and in some cases even 40).

The creation of these performances is a complex process that requires not only passion but also varied skills, as well as the willingness to invest, for the benefit of the group, the *freguesia*, and the island, time inevitably taken away from other activities and leisure pursuits.

Each performance requires musicians able to play different instruments (preferably more than one) and to execute simple, largely codified choreographic movements, which nonetheless must be performed in coordination. Actors are needed—confident and with stage presence—who, in addition to memorising lines, have the communication skills and improvisational ability to engage the audience.

There are also the authors of the scripts—containing passages in verse—and of the music: they may be from the same village and part of the performing group, or specialists working for many groups, writing new scripts and music each year or adapting music and lyrics from previous years.

Hélio Costa, one of the legendary figures of Terceira's Carnival—after whom the Carnival Museum of Lajes is named—wrote as many as 1305 performances in his lifetime, some also for the Azorean diaspora communities.

We must not forget those who work on the preparation of the numerous, often elaborate and imaginative costumes and stage sets, nor those responsible for stage equipment and theatre management—a demanding and delicate task for anyone with theatrical experience.

Invisible work also includes the hosting of groups arriving at the theatres to perform: from organising the parking of minibuses to setting up the *mesa*—a table with food and drink, mostly homemade, traditionally—prepared by the women of the *freguesia* together with the local council or the leaders of the Casa do Povo.

This *mesa*, with which each *freguesia* and theatre honours and thanks the groups, plays an important role in community life as it measures organisational ability, willingness to commit, culinary skills, and, in some ways, the economic strength of each community. "Taste this wine. It's special. You won't find it anywhere else, because it's produced only here in this *freguesia*" is a recurring phrase that anyone lucky enough to be admitted to the room reserved for the *mesa* will hear repeated in almost every *freguesia*.

There is also political and administrative organisation of the performance, as well as of the time and space of the festival, which includes continuous negotiation between groups, their spokespersons, *freguesia* councils, and the two municipalities to secure funding, agree on the touring of performances, and determine the order of appearance in different theatres, and so on.

The performances are the result of largely invisible work carried out before and during Carnival: in homes, rehearsal rooms, the offices of *freguesia* councils, Casas do Povo, and municipal buildings; on stage, backstage, in reserved rooms, in theatre bars and catering areas, and in the spaces outside theatres.

This work also has an embedded time dimension that is largely invisible: preparatory meetings, discussions, rehearsals, and, finally, the hectic Carnival days when groups tour the island from mid-afternoon until late at night performing their shows.

We must not forget the feelings, emotions, and other intangible aspects that accompany and give meaning to this commitment: anticipation, joy, satisfaction, fatigue, nervousness, fun, pride, and competition.

All this, as we have seen, involves a significant number of people and is indicative of the symbolic importance and experiential centrality of this Carnival.

If theatre, to use an expression by Riccioni (2022), can be a collective social practice "which weaves the meaning of the territory, people and generations" and, through a "continuous rethinking" of the community's values, practices, and events, "contributes to creating meaningfulness and consolidating cohabitation", then the Carnival of Terceira certainly fulfils this role to the highest degree.

Its dual nature—participatory and ritual—expressing the community and its history, makes it a living element of cultural heritage that, for the moment, is able to accompany, with the smile of Carnival, the community through a complicated present and into the uncharted lands of the future. A Carnival that has managed to absorb postmodernity without being swallowed by it, and which shows that tradition can still have a role.

References

Almeida, O. T. (2008). Comunidades portuguesas nos Estados Unidos: identidade, assimilaçâo, aculuraçâo. In M. Lages & A. T. de Matos (Eds.), *Portugal: percursos de interculturalidade* (pp. 339–422). Alto Comissariado para a Imigraçâo e Diálogo Intercultural.

Bachtin, M. M. (1941). *Rabelais and His World*. Indiana University Press.

Baganha, M. I. (1990). *Portuguese emigration to the United States, 1820–1930*. Garland Publishing.

Bretão, J. N. (1998). *As Danças do Entrudo. Uma Festa do Povo: Teatro Popular da Ilha Terceira* (Vol. I). Direcção Regional da Cultura.

Caretos de Podence. (2025). Entrudo Chocalheiro—2026. Eventos. https://www.caretosdepodence.pt/node/294

Caro Baroja, J. (1979). *El carnaval: análisis histórico-cultural*. Taurus.

Cellini, R. (2011). Is UNESCO recognition effective in fostering tourism? A comment on Yang, Lin and Han. *Tourism Management, 32*(2), 452–454.

Corbisiero, F., & Monaco, S. (2025). *Sociologia del turismo. Tra terra, acqua, aria e fuoco*. Utet.

Cordeiro, G. I., & Formato, G. (2024). Azorean-American resilience in Camberville: A visual approach to a vernacular landscape in a gentrified neighborhood. In S. Lakić, P. Pereira & G. Í. Cordeiro (Eds.), *The Everydayness of Cities in Transition Micro Approaches to Material and Social Dimensions of Change* (pp. 121–154). Palgrave Macmillan.

Corvo, P. (2007). *Turisti e felici? Il turismo tra benessere e fragilità*. Edizioni di Comunità.

Cuccia, T., Guccio, C., & Rizzo, I. (2016). The effects of UNESCO world heritage list inscription on tourism destinations performance in Italian regions. *Economic Modelling, 53*(C), 494–508.

Duarte, L. F. (2010). O Carnaval na ilha Terceira. *Comunicaçâo & Cultura, 10*, 87–100.
Enes, C. (1989). O Carnaval angrense no 1° terço do Século XX. *Boletim do Instituto Histórico da Ilha Terceira, 47*, 291–365.
Fabre, D. (1992). *Carnaval ou la fête à l'envers*. Gallimard.
Falcâo Mendes, A. (2018). Danças, Bailinhos e Comédias do Carnavl da Ilha Terceira. *CulturAçores. Revista da Cultura, 9*, 21–25.
Fonseca, J. (2025, February 25). *O Carnaval da Ilha Terceira na construçâo da cidadania ativa e crítica* [Conference presentation]. Simpósio Carnaval Teatro e Sociedade entre os palcos e a escola. Universidade dos Açores, Ponta Delgada, Portugal.
Hawkes, J. (2001). *The fourth pillar of sustainability: Culture's essential role in public planning*. Cultural Development Network and Part of University Press.
Huang, C. H., Tsaur, J. R., & Yang, C. H. (2012). Does world heritage list really induce more tourists? Evidence from Macau. *Tourism Management, 33*(6), 1450–1457.
IPDT – Instituto de Turismo. (2020). *Plano estratégico e de marketing do turismo dos Acores*. IPDT.
Langman, L. (2008). Carnivalization: The Body and the Liminal. From the Flaneur to the Urban Primitive. In B. M. Pirani & I. Varga (Eds.), *The New Boundaries Between Bodies and Technologies* (pp. 55–90). Cambridge Scholars Publishing.
Leal, J. (1994). *As festas do Espírito Santo nos Açores. Um estudo de Antropologia Social*. Dom Quixote.
Leal, J. (2017). *O culto do divino. Migrações e transformações*. Edições 70.
Lusa. (2025, August 5). Regiâo deve definir limites de crescimento do turismo. Açoriano Oriental, 7.
MacCannell, D. (1973). Staged authenticity: Arrangements of social space in tourist settings. *American Journal of Sociology, 79*(3), 589–603.
Marcelli, A. M. (2023). *Charting the Entrudo: Ecopedagogy of cultural heritage in the European outermost region of the Azores*. Pensa Multimedia.
Marcelli, A. M., Sousa, F., Fonseca, J., Sampaio da Silva, L., Melotti, M., & Goulart Costa, S. (2022). The unknown carnival of Terceira Island (Azores, Portugal): Community, heritage, and identity on stage. *Sustainability, 14*(20), 13250. https://doi.org/10.3390/su142013250
Martins, C. (2025). Olé toiro Terceira. Bailinho Amigos do Carnaval de Amigos de São Brás. Terceira (Portugal).
MatrizPCI. (2016). Danças, Bailinhos e Comédias do Carnaval da Ilha Terceira. *Inventário Nacional do Patrimonio Cultural Imaterial.* Ficha de Património *Imaterial* [n° de inventário: INPCI_2020_002]. https://matrizpci.patrimoniocultural.gov.pt/InventarioNacional/DetalheFicha/500?dirPesq=3
Melotti, M. (2010). Oltre il Carnevale. Maschere e postmodernità. In P. Sisto & P. Totaro (Eds.), *Il Carnevale e il Mediterraneo. Tradizioni, riti e maschere del Mezzogiorno d'Italia* (pp. 57–88). Progedit.
Melotti, M. (2019). *Carnevalizzazione e società postmoderna. Maschere, linguaggi, paure*. Progedit.
Melotti, M. (2025). Taormina. Sguardo turistico e cristallizzazione dello spazio urbano. *Quaderni di Sociologia, 97*(1), 165-190.
Melotti, M. (2026). Terceira and beyond. Carnivals, globalization and contemporary society. In *Anuário do Carnaval Terceirense*. Separata do Boletim do instituto Histórico da Ilha Terceira, 1 [In press].
Município de Macedo de Cavaleiros. (2018, October 10). Sugestâo de fim-de-semana. Facebook. https://www.facebook.com/cm.macedodecavaleiros/photos/sugest%C3%A3o-de-fim-de-semanaos-caretos-representam-imagens-diab%C3%B3licas-e-misteriosas/2057997607596595/
Olson, D. (2025). The Carnivalesque character of Aristophanic comedy. [Conference presentation]. Simpósio Carnaval Teatro e Sociedade entre os palcos e a escola. Universidade dos Açores, Ponta Delgada, Portugal.

Paltrinieri, R. (2022). Theatre at university as a way to increase the sense. In I. Riccioni (Ed.), *(2002). Theatre(s) and public sphere in a global and digital society. Volume 1. Theoretical explorations* (pp. 41–48). Brill.

Riccioni, I. (Ed.). (2022). *Theatre(s) and public sphere in a global and digital society (Vol. 1). Theoretical explorations*. Brill.

Rocha, G. P. N., Ferreira, E., & Mendes, D. (2011). *Between Worlds. Emigration and Return to the Azores*. Government of the Azores.

Soini, K., & Birkeland, I. (2014). Exploring the scientific discourse on cultural sustainability. *Geoforum, 51*, 213–223.

Visit Portugal. (n.d.). *The Caretos of Podence*. https://www.visitportugal.com/en/node/139277

Part III
Actors

Chapter 10
A Theatre for the City: The Case of the Prose Seasons at the Donizetti Theatre in Bergamo

Maria Grazia Panigada

Don't expect the theatre to satisfy the habits of its audience, but to change them

Bertold Brecht

Bergamo is divided into two parts: the historic upper town, perched on top of a hill and enclosed by imposing walls built during the rule of the Venetian Republic in the sixteenth century, and the lower town. It was here, in the heart of the latter, that a grand theatre was inaugurated in 1791, commissioned by a wealthy merchant Bortolo Riccardi. A few years later, a fire severely damaged much of the structure, which was rebuilt into what stands today: a theatre with one of the largest auditoriums in Italy, featuring three tiers of boxes and two tiers of galleries, which can accommodate up to 1200 spectators. From being owned by a single private individual, the theatre in 1895 transitioned to a citizens' corporation before becoming municipal property. Throughout its history, the theatre has always remained active, having hosted notable artists such as Ermete Novelli and Maria Callas on its stage.

Between 2018 and 2020, the Donizetti theatre (since 1897 named after the great composer from Bergamo) has undergone an extensive restoration and architectural renovation. Today it is a modern theatre in line with the latest safety regulations, while having kept its nineteenth-century charm intact.

Even the "Upper town" in Bergamo has its own theatre, the *Teatro Sociale* ("Social theatre"): a true gem nestled among mediaeval buildings and narrow streets, where its facade blends seamlessly with the neighbouring buildings. It was built from a design by Leopoldo Pollack, among the most celebrated architects of the Neoclassical period, and was inaugurated in 1808.

The building remained an active performance venue until 1932, when activity began to slowly decline, with the space being used only sporadically for performances and exhibitions. This phase ended in 2006, when a joint initiative of the City

M. G. Panigada (✉)
Teatro Donizetti, Bergamo, Italy

P. Corvo, I. Riccioni (eds.), *Theatre and Quality of Life*, Social Indicators Research Series 91, https://doi.org/10.1007/978-3-032-09731-6_10

Council and the Superintendency launched an extensive restoration project. In 2009, the completely renovated theatre officially reopened its doors to the public. With its elegant French-style oval design, Teatro Sociale features 82 boxes arranged across three tiers. A structural reinforcement plan was also introduced for the gallery in order to make it easily accessible to the public in the future. Currently, the Teatro Sociale has a capacity of about 500 seats.

Both the Donizetti and the Sociale theatres are the property of the Municipality of Bergamo. In 2014, the Teatro Donizetti Foundation was established to manage both venues and oversee all related cultural activities. In particular, beyond the prose season, the foundation organizes an important Jazz Festival and the Donizetti Opera Festival, entirely dedicated to the works of composer Gaetano Donizetti. The program also includes operettas, concerts, and other composers' operas. Since 1962, the Donizetti theatre has also hosted every year the International Piano Festival alongside the *Teatro Grande* of Brescia.

Bergamo, with a population of 120,000 inhabitants and over a million residents in its province, is a mid-sized Italian city located just 56 kilometres from Milan, a metropolis hosting more than 40 theatres (excluding provincial ones).

For this reason, it is remarkable that in 2024 alone the Donizetti foundation has welcomed about 100,000 spectators across its two theatres, registered more than 7500 subscribers across its various programmes, and involved more than 20,000 young people in its educational projects.

Particularly noteworthy is the prose theatre section, which has become a case study in the national panorama, for both attendance numbers and audience quality. The numbers speak for themselves: attendance has consistently grown for several years, especially after the forced hiatus due to the Covid 19 pandemic that dramatically affected this geographical area. Unlike in many other Italian cities, where audience numbers declined after theatres reopened, there was no drop in attendance, but citizens immediately re-inhabited the theatre.

To get an idea of the attendance trend we can compare the current season with the previous two: over the past 3 years, the subscription renewal rate has remained exceptionally high, between 94 and 97%. From this we can obtain a first data point: the high level of audience satisfaction. Yet, even with such a solid base, attendance has continued to rise every year. The number of annual subscribers to the prose season grew from 4691 in 2022/2023 to 5181 the following year, reaching 5731 in the 2024/2025 season. This increase of over 1000 subscribers in just two seasons has led to the introduction of an additional performance, bringing the total to eight showings per production. This decision was taken also to answer adequately, on top of the subscriptions, to the increasingly high demand for single tickets, which often the theatre cannot accommodate due to fully selling out.

The Theatre of the City: *or Rather*, How Do You Programme for a Theatre?

Programming a theatre begins with watching theatre. It may seem like an obvious statement, but in reality, it really is not. In Italy, only a handful of artistic directors travel all across the peninsula to directly select productions for their seasons. More often, programming decisions are based on factors other than direct viewing—such as partnerships among established theatres for major co-productions, reciprocal agreements to ensure their production gets good touring opportunities, or the presence on stage of recognized and famous actors.

Personally, I would not be able to program without first sitting among the audience, suspending all judgements and focusing solely on the experience before me.

A programming style rooted in expertise demands a full range of acquired skills and knowledge, gained through nearly three decades of work in the field. Yet, each time the lights go down and a performance begins, that knowledge and those skills are tested anew.

Only during the pandemic did I have to rely on watching full videos of the performances, but it was an obligatory choice due to the current events, and an extremely difficult one for me. I believe that on paper, or in videos, a show is not entirely assessable: only direct viewing allows one to understand the staging as a whole, not only the direction and interpretation, but also the sets, the lighting, and the music…

Going around visiting theatres means meeting the artists, getting to know what they plan on working on in the future, and creating possibilities for collaborations on side projects outside of the current season.

Each time I am evaluating a show, I also try to envision how it might be received by Bergamo's audience, and what possibilities it might offer for deeper engagement beyond the performance itself.

My approach seeks a balance—programming productions that will surely be enjoyed while also taking some risks, daring audiences to dive into new territories of poetics, staging, and dramaturgy.

Every year, I receive around 300 show proposals, of which I select approximately 90 to personally attend. From these, I make a final selection of 20 to 25 titles. Depending on the season, I ultimately program between 14 and 18 productions, adjusting to the calendar's needs. This varies for example for special sections or single events—for example, when we have dedicated a segment to historical themes.

Direct relationships with artists and producers also make it possible to know in advance, for example, what new show a director is starting to work on. This allows Teatro Donizetti to showcase new works, sometimes anticipating neighboring venues. In such cases, as an artistic director, I gather as much information as possible about the production in advance. For example, I request scripts to read, attend rehearsals if the show is already being staged, and engage in discussions with the creative team—discussing with the production team the choices they have made and how they plan to tour the work, dialoguing back and forth both with the actors and the director.

When selecting performances, I do not prioritize commercial appeal or the presence of well-known actors, such as those from television, to guarantee easy success. That approach might bring a few successful nights, but it would not foster long-term audience engagement. Furthermore, as a civic theatre, our mission is to contribute to cultural enrichment, not just entertainment.

The strong audience numbers in recent years are the result of a decade-long commitment to quality—one that has sometimes required difficult choices, but has ultimately built trust. Today, Bergamo's audience knows they can rely on our offerings, even if they are unfamiliar with the playwright's or actors' names.

The programming is divided into two main sections: the Prose Season at Teatro Donizetti and *Altri percorsi* ("Alternative routes"), which primarily takes place at Teatro Sociale. Altri Percorsi was born in 1980 through the vision of Benvenuto Cuminetti, a professor of theatre history and the soul of the flourishing of prose in Bergamo. His innovation was to introduce some experimentation in the programming of a municipal theatre—making Teatro Donizetti the first historical theatre in Italy to systematically include research theatre in its playbill.

When curating this section, it is important for me to give spectators, on the one hand, the opportunity to follow certain artists over time, and on the other hand, to include each year companies that are being hosted for the first time. I firmly believe that Italy's theatre scene holds remarkable talent among the new generations, yet emerging artists often struggle to find the space they deserve. This is why theatre festivals in Italy play a crucial role, providing professionals like myself with the opportunity to discover fresh voices and innovative works in a few days—helping to ensure that the "new" theatre finds its audience.

While there are a few production experiences undertaken by the prose sector (the Donizetti Foundation produces three or four stagings of Donizetti operas each year), each of them has allowed us to discover the immense potential of in-house productions—something that we hope in the future will become a constant.

A few notable examples highlight this potential. One of the latest productions, *Iliade. Il gioco degli dèi* ("Iliade. Game of the gods") is a co-production with a private theatre (Marco Balsamo's Teatro Nuovo), a national theatre (the *Pergola—Teatro della Toscana*) and a civic theatre (*Teatro Stabile del Friuli-Venezia Giulia*). Created for Bergamo-Brescia 2023 Italian Capital of Culture, the production completed 150 performances in 2 years alone, and is likely to go on a third year of touring, bringing the Donizetti Foundation's name to audiences around Italy.

Beyond the stage, the production also served as an educational tool: local high school students created a documentary about the *Iliade*, capturing the creative process through rehearsal footage and interviews—not only with the protagonists on stage, but also with the many professionals working behind the scenes. This show was particularly well-suited for such an in-depth exploration, as it is rooted in figurative theatre, offering insight into the entire creative process, from initial sketches to the construction of the characters-mannequins and masks. At the same time, we offered adult audiences a series of in-depth events on the theme of the show.

Another example of excellent touring is *Per te* ("For you"), a show produced with the Finzi Pasca company thanks to a collaboration with a technical sponsor based in the Clay Paky territory (the world's leading brand in professional lighting systems). The show has toured the world from Hungary to Mexico, from Canada to the prestigious Brisbane Festival in Australia.

We then focused on small productions related to the sphere of research theatre, such as *Ivan*, made with the ATIR company, which was presented for two seasons in a row at the Piccolo Teatro in Milan, or *Accabadora*, created with director Veronica Cruciani and developed by sharing the creative process with author Michela Murgia. The show premiered in 2018 at the Teatro Sociale, and is still touring. There was also a little gem, *Egloga XI*, produced by the Anagoor company. All these shows were opportunities to create insights, opportunities for reflection and study.

Increasing the Audience: *or Rather*, a Choice of Public Development and Teamwork

I never thought that the overriding goal of my artistic direction was to increase the audience: this has always been for me a consequence of good practice. When sitting in the audience of a show, if it is visible that the audience is happy because they recognize a TV star, or laughs at some silly joke, it could be easy to think of bringing that show to Bergamo just to easily fill the theatre, but it is other criteria that guide me. The audience must be educated. To educate is a verb deriving from the Latin *exducere*, meaning to lead outside, to bring beyond, to make the unexpected known. In this sense it is important for me that the audience meets the different languages of which theatre is composed.

For example, in 2008 our bill featured *Nebbia*, produced by the Canadian *Cirque Eloize*. The first performances did not go particularly well, but by word of mouth, on the last day we had a long line in front of the box office. Since then, periodically, our season hosts circus-theatre shows, which are still rare in the Italian theatre scene, but our audiences are now familiar with these kinds of shows, and wait for them. We are recognized in this field as one of the most important theatres in Italy, which is why we were able to bring in 2015 *La Verità* ("The Truth") by Compagnia Finzi Pasca in the version with the large original stage tarpaulin (fifteen metres by nine) made by Salvador Dalì.

The season is built by mixing various ingredients to intrigue and to experiment with the public. I like to think of the drama season as a place where people go to gain something: an emotion, an encounter, sometimes even an annoyance, but still always looking for something that can raise new questions inside them, a place to share with others a time of listening, and looking. A place where people with different stories, different ages, and different thoughts, can go and, for the time of the performance, sit together. And every time something incredible happens, if we really let ourselves get involved (by finally turning off our cell phones), time becomes suspended in other places and times, and the story on stage offers itself to us, unique and unrepeatable, because the conditions of a live performance will never be the exact same.

Some prefer classical auteur theatre, others are drawn to contemporary drama, some want to be distracted, and others crave intellectual depth. Yet, every choice must adhere to a standard of quality—one that often focuses on themes of contemporaneity, human relationships across distant social contexts and historical periods, but all united by an inquiry that transcends the contingent to embrace complexity. This is, after all, the essence of theatre: a space where we enter certainly of our present, but keep our minds and hearts open to encountering the unknown. It lasts only for the duration of the performance, but perhaps, in that fleeting time, it offers us the chance to relativize, question, and deepen our thinking.

The audience is constantly increasing, also thanks to the side projects and meetings that foster the involvement of younger generations: the Donizetti theatre has become an ever-growing community, always becoming more inclusive and welcoming. The troupes that we host tell us that ours is a theatre where they can breathe in the skills of the workers and the welcoming atmosphere of the staff employed here. But, above all, they are surprised by the audience: they feel, as they perform, they are in front of competent, respectful spectators who truly know how to listen. That is another reason why the choice of each show requires great responsibility and must be taken carefully and precisely.

In the same way, something that requires great attention is the involvement of individuals who, without our help, would hardly be able to access the theatre. For example, over the years we have collaborated with the local prison, with first reception facilities, with support centres for those struggling with addiction or housing emergencies. For the under-nineteens, we have created a subscription to the *Altri Percorsi* season for a very low price that includes an introductory meeting before the shows, moments of discussions with the actors and directors and group sharing of the experience.

But if the choice of titles is mine, the credit for the Donizetti Foundation's achievement in the prose sector belongs to an entire work team and to an atmosphere of mutual cooperation. Let's think about how important some professions are for the relationship with the reception of a theatre, such as the box office staff, or the theatre hall staff. The former who listens to everyone's needs, recommends seats, suggests the most suitable shows, patiently recognizes and solves the many small problems of the audience. The latter, the ushers, who open the doors of the theatre and welcome the audience, are guides and gatekeepers who coordinate access logistics, are at the disposal of the spectators, and ensure the optimal unfolding of the show so that the live performance can be properly enjoyed.

Similarly, for guest companies, it is essential to find concierge staff who welcomes, responds to different needs, and creates a family-like environment, but also to be supported by stage workers who are not only competent, but also willing to help solve problems that may arise during a stage assembly. And then there are those who do hidden work that neither the public, nor the companies, see. These are all the colleagues who follow the administration, make the contracts, take care of the paperwork, and follow the press office and the communication.

These are all different professional profiles who invest a lot of care and commitment in their work. I am convinced that this is what truly makes a season beautiful.

Education, *or Rather* at the Heart of the Theatre

The Donizetti theatre is a civic theatre, and as such its priority is the education and active participation of young citizens. For this reason, the Donizetti Foundation has activated an in-house office dedicated to Educational Services. This office plans, compares, and verifies every educational project it proposes and implements. These, too, are good public development practices because, by getting young boys and girls excited about the drama theatre, they bring younger audiences to the theatre. But this is only a consequence of what our priorities are: to make the Bergamo theatre a place of meeting for the community, a place to reflect, a place in which shows can each time become valuable opportunities for discussion and deepening through communal paths and meetings.

When we talk with the teenagers involved in our projects, a hidden, intimate aspect emerges: that thanks to our projects, they have begun to pay more attention to the reality that surrounds them, or to the history that precedes them. In other words, we have generated in them a change towards a better listening, towards a more conscious reflection on themselves and others.

Over time, through these projects, a structured work team has formed within the Educational Services, composed of workers specialized and trained with different skills, ranging from young adults trained at our own theatre school to key figures from the civil community. The collaboration between professionals of different backgrounds enables us to design projects that integrate seamlessly into the different school curricula, and can be adapted to the needs of specialized high schools.

A characteristic feature of our projects, which has emerged even more after the pandemic, is the importance of listening to young voices as an indispensable element, not only for youth engagement, but also as a resource for our own institution and knowledge. In more complex projects, teenage participants are called to take on active responsibility and make their voices heard, which is further enhanced through the Foundation's communication and social channels.

Projects for schools are always structured around one or more shows taken from the drama season or the Altri Percorsi section.

On the one hand, there are workshops linked to the viewing of classical screenings, from Shakespeare to Goldoni, from Aeschylus to De Filippo. In these cases, the projects are aimed at giving interpretations of the show to allow the students to experience the dramaturgy starting from their own experience. The text should interrogate them personally, having them take on a critical gaze and allowing them to experience the theatre as an experience that directly concerns them. For example, different versions of the same script are screened before the show, comparing different directors and styles, to give the students hints on how to detect the important aspects of staging, such as the lighting aspect, or the choice of sounds and music.

On the other hand, we offer a range of projects connected to new dramaturgy and productions by young companies. In these initiatives, the role of theatre within the civil community takes on even greater significance, becoming a central place for dialogue on contemporary issues. In recent years, we have used theatre to foster reflections on justice, the environment, social rights, and diversity. However, it is crucial that these discussions do not remain abstract. That is why we actively involve local organizations, grounding theoretical reflections in real-life experiences. For example, we have collaborated with communities supporting unaccompanied foreign minors, with "public hotels" assisting homeless individuals in housing reintegration, as well as neighbourhood initiatives such as social gardens or organizations tackling food waste.

A special focus has to be given to performances related to historical themes, where we aim to engage students as active and responsible participants. Over the years, we have conducted extensive research through staged plays on the theme of the Resistance during World War II. In collaboration with the ISREC (the Bergamo Institute for the Resistance History and Contemporary Resistance), we have ensured that each project includes a dedicated section on teaching students how to conduct historical research. By working directly with local sources and archives, students not only gain a deeper understanding of history but also develop critical thinking skills, learning how to analyse reality through the lens of the past.

Emphasizing the significance of these historical themes does not detract from the theatrical experience. Instead, it enriches it—allowing for a deeper exploration of theatrical language in its various forms and a greater appreciation of different artistic styles.

The Donizetti theatre Educational Services offer programs for all secondary schools in the city and province: high schools, technical institutes, and professional schools. Over time, we have recognized the value of fostering exchanges between students from diverse academic backgrounds. When logistics allow, these moments of interaction create opportunities to intertwine different perspectives and enhance learning through shared experiences.

Another key focus of the Donizetti Foundation's education programs are courses preparing students for theatrical professions. Among these, *Progetto Young* is a three-year acting course accessible through a selective process. Under the guidance of Fabio Comana, students develop techniques, experience ensemble work, and are encouraged to cultivate their own theatrical style. Throughout the year, participants also benefit from the insights of artists featured in the theatre's seasonal programming. Over the past decade, several of our graduates have been accepted into Italy's most prestigious theatre academies and are now established professionals. Others have transitioned directly into local theatre companies or founded their own. In addition to the acting course, we alternate between offerings in playwriting and stagehand training. Every year, we also provide professional orientation courses in lighting and sound design, led by the theatre's technical staff. At the end of each program, students from various courses collaborate to create a performance, which is then presented to the city.

It is precisely this commitment to education—without diminishing our many offerings for adult audiences—that has allowed the Donizetti theatre to establish itself as a true *house of culture*: a dynamic space, a hub of multidisciplinary exchange, and a vital centre for artistic growth.

Chapter 11
Confession of a Director

Carlo Roncaglia

The Role of the Director Today

To speak about the role of the director today means, at least for me, to recount a personal journey. I can't do it without starting from my own experience: that of a man of theatre who has lived the stage in many ways—as a director, artistic director, actor, and spectator—and who continues to live it every day. My entire professional life has revolved around the theatre.

Doing theatre is not merely a job: it is a choice rooted in a deep passion, which over time has become a profession, with all the responsibilities, challenges, and satisfactions that come with it. It's certainly a difficult path, but one full of inspiration, encounters, and possibilities.

In Italy, the director began to take on a central role especially from the 1960s onwards. Before that, the heart of the theatre was the actor: leading actors at the head of their own companies, star performers, a theatrical "star system" that has almost entirely disappeared today. The shift to director-driven theatre marked a turning point: the focus moved from performance to project, from acting to an overarching vision. Bringing a text to the stage—whether classic or contemporary—became an act of rewriting. Whether subtle or radical, it doesn't matter: it is always a form of active interpretation. A creative process.

In this sense, the director becomes a second author. Some major figures have left an indelible mark on twentieth- and early twenty-first-century theatre: Peter Brook, Eimuntas Nekrosius, Peter Stein, Anatolij Vasiliev, Robert Wilson, and in Italy, Giorgio Strehler, Luca Ronconi, Giancarlo Cobelli, Cesare Lievi, and Massimo Castri. Very different figures, yet all capable of leaving a profound imprint. Personally, I've been lucky not only to see many of their productions, but also to

C. Roncaglia (✉)
Accademia dei Folli, Torino, Italy
e-mail: info@accademiadeifolli.com

P. Corvo, I. Riccioni (eds.), *Theatre and Quality of Life*, Social Indicators Research Series 91, https://doi.org/10.1007/978-3-032-09731-6_11

come into direct contact with some of them. Ronconi, for example, was my teacher at the Teatro Stabile School in Turin, and his approach to directing deeply influenced my perspective.

If we had to explain to someone unfamiliar with theatre what it really is, we wouldn't speak of its "magic". We'd say something simpler: it's someone saying something to someone else, in a certain place and at a certain time. That's all. Theatre happens in the relationship between those who act and those who watch. It is a form of presence.

But even director-driven theatre, over time, has revealed its limitations. The strong sense of authorship that once brought innovation and energy has, in some cases, become self-referential. Productions have grown increasingly complex—and sometimes inaccessible—to the point of excluding the audience rather than involving them. The distance has widened. Theatre, once a vibrant dialogue, has at times turned into a stylistic exercise. And that's a problem, because theatre doesn't work without relationship. It can't be reduced to form. It can't be passively received: it must be lived.

In recent years, we've seen a turn towards more direct, almost confrontational forms of theatre—productions that often resemble stand-up comedy more than traditional drama. It's no longer even narrative theatre in the sense that Dario Fo, Marco Paolini, or Ascanio Celestini gave it: it's something new, that has completely lost the fourth wall and often, too, its emotional depth.

I still believe in that symbolic space that separates the stage from the audience. Not as a wall, but as a threshold. It's there that the possibility of entering the story is built.

After more than 25 years of work, I believe that directing should no longer be a showcase for proving how clever one is. I've learned to let go of the need to create just for the sake of it. Today, I feel my task is to make what I put on stage understandable, effective, and necessary.

Direction must serve communication. It must reach today's audience—an audience accustomed to fast rhythms, polished visuals, and quick content. Theatre, however, asks for time, attention, and listening. And that pact must be renewed every time.

I believe theatre must return to being something essential. Not for everyone, perhaps, but for many. It must be accessible, engaging, and beautiful. Just as it was in ancient Athens, when even slaves could attend theatrical contests. Theatre had a public function—and it's that function, I believe, that we must rediscover.

Theatre as Social Action

I have always smiled, with a certain sense of wonder, when I hear someone say, "I do social theatre", as if there could be a form of theatre that isn't social. In truth, every kind of theatre involves a social dimension. Simply gathering people together in the same place, at the same time, to share an experience is, in itself, a social act. In fact, it is perhaps one of the oldest and most essential social acts we can perform.

By its very nature, theatre happens in the present. It happens here and now. It comes into being at the exact moment it is experienced by an audience. This makes it, whether we like it or not, a lens through which we view the contemporary world. Even when staging a classic—be it *Richard III*, *The Cherry Orchard*, *Right You Are (If You Think So)*, *A Doll's House*, *The Mistress of the Inn*, or *Medea*—we are doing it today, with today's perspective, for today's audience. We engage with it through the filter of the present. And the spectator, in turn, adds a second filter, that of their own sensitivity, inevitably shaped by the time they live in. The distance between a contemporary audience and a spectator at Epidaurus attending the ancient theatrical contests is vast. Yet it is precisely this distance that makes every theatrical gesture contemporary.

Yes, theatre has a social function. Yes, it is a tool to question the present, to take stock of where we are and where we want to go. And yes, it is a shared process: it's not only those on stage who create it, but also those who watch. It is a form of assembly, with its own particular rules, of course, but with a very clear purpose: to focus our gaze on the contemporary.

When I read a script and begin to imagine how to bring it to the stage, I inevitably start from today. *Richard III*, for instance, speaks to me differently now than it did 10 years ago. I read it through the lens of today's thoughts, fears, and images. The production is born from that perspective. Theatre and real-time coincide: reading and acting are both anchored in the present. And it is this bond that makes theatre necessary. Useful. Social.

At the same time, theatre is also a form of transfiguration. It does not seek realism. On the contrary, it is precisely the lack of realism that allows for abstraction, evocation, and exploration. The distance from the real world enables us to dig deeper, to represent not merely individual cases, but archetypes. The universality of theatre is born from this: from its ability to touch the symbolic, to narrate the deep roots of things.

There is another dimension that I feel very close to me, both as a director and as a spectator: the idea of theatre that doesn't offer answers, but opens up questions. That leaves space for doubt, for unresolved questions. Just as it happened in Greek theatre. Take *Prometheus*: it raises an issue that remains unresolved even today. Does humankind have the right to possess technology? Perhaps yes. But are we capable of using it wisely? Or will we be overwhelmed by it?

Every era responds differently to the same questions. My generation grew up reading science fiction stories that now seem like news reports. We are living through an incredible acceleration. And yet theatre—even though it works through symbols, myths, and ancient figures—remains anchored to the present. It always speaks to today, even when it tells stories written 2000 years ago.

This becomes evident every time we approach a classic. Even in the most philological productions, even when trying to reproduce it "as it was back then", something inevitably changes. The stage changes, the context changes, the audience changes. And so, inevitably, the meaning changes as well.

And finally, perhaps the simplest and most powerful thing: theatre does not exist without an audience. It is the only art form that requires at least one person in front of it. You can play music for yourself, write for yourself, sculpt or hang your painting in your living room. But no actor can perform alone. Without an external gaze, there is no theatre. This once again confirms how profoundly social, communal, and participatory an art form it is. It never belongs solely to the artist. It is a shared gesture. And it is a gesture that takes place in the present.

Theatre and Quality of Life (for Those Who Create It and for the Audience)

Talking about theatre and quality of life means, first and foremost, asking what it means to live by doing theatre. For those who create it, of course, but also for those who experience it as an audience. And perhaps starting with those who work in it is the most direct way to approach the question.

There are at least two aspects that seem fundamental to me. The first is that working in theatre inevitably means engaging with beauty, literature, philosophy, psychology, and sociology. It's a job that forces you to stay curious, to ask questions, to seek answers. It constantly puts you in relation with others, with other people's thoughts, with other people's feelings. It compels you to observe, to dig deep. It's a profession that continually enriches you. And this, in itself, is already a privilege. It's not a given to be able to make a living doing something that demands you to think, to listen, to grow. Something that often stems from a deep passion and that—sometimes—manages to become a real job.

Then there's another element, perhaps less poetic but just as significant: theatre is one of the few professions that, besides a pay check, also gives you applause. There is public recognition. Of course, it's part of the theatrical convention, but it remains a powerful moment. It's as if someone were saying to you: "I saw your work, I listened to it, it moved me". It's a sign that arrives immediately, directly, and is shared. And at certain moments, it repays many hardships.

That's why I've always thought we are lucky. It's a job that forces you to study, to update yourself, to sharpen your tools. You can't just repeat yourself. You can't afford to stand still. It's a craft that can't be done on autopilot. It keeps you awake.

I often talk about this in the training courses I conduct in different fields, including the corporate world. The role of the director is particularly interesting to analyse because it combines creativity and leadership. A director must make decisions and also mediate between different visions, manage time and resources, listen to the actors' energy, and build a shared path. They need method, empathy, and vision. It's a role that requires a balance between craftsmanship and art. And this is especially true in theatre.

Craftsmanship is the part you can control: the technique, the skill, the precision. Art, on the other hand, is that elusive thing that you never know if it will come. That moment of grace, that drop of splendour—to borrow the words of De André—that you chase your whole life. You cannot seize it, but you can prepare yourself for it. You can train yourself to recognize it, to make room for it. Craftsmanship is practiced; art is awaited.

So yes, theatre has a huge impact on the quality of life of those who create it. I feel fortunate to be able to say that: it's my profession. And in my case, the boundary between work and passion is often difficult to draw. Where one ends, the other begins.

But it's not all simple. There is also a downside. Those who work in theatre often live under constant tension: toward a goal, toward a result, toward recognition. The bar is always raised. You achieve something? You want to achieve something greater. You reach a milestone? It already feels surpassed. It's a form of constant dissatisfaction, a search that never stops.

When I graduated from the Scuola del Teatro Stabile di Torino in 1997, my goal was very concrete: to succeed in turning theatre into a profession. To be able to make a living from it. After a few years, with effort, I succeeded. I had founded a company—Accademia dei Folli—and from there, I built a path. But it has been a constant process of setting new goals: working, yes, but living well. Living well, yes, but also being recognized. Being recognized, yes, but not just within a niche. And so on.

Then there are difficult moments. Periods of stagnation when you feel stuck. Frustration, discouragement, and that feeling of no longer being useful. Sometimes it's not even a real failure, but you feel it nonetheless. Then you get back up. You start moving again. You invent something new. It happens. And it happens often.

In this sense, theatre resembles life a lot. It is made of ups and downs, of crises and restarts. It is a mirror of existence, for better or worse. And it forces you to live it intensely, without holding back.

Another aspect to consider, however, concerns the context we live in. In Italy, working in theatre is still very difficult. There is no real system that supports, accompanies, or values it. There is a lack of a strong cultural vision. Clear training paths for many theatre professions are missing. Yes, there are academies, and some have been recognized at university level, but there are no professional schools for all the roles involved in theatre production.

It's strange, considering the history we have, our tradition, and the artistic richness we inherit. And yet theatre here has never really been considered an economic sector, an investment. Unlike in other countries, such as France or those in the Anglo-Saxon world, where culture is also seen as a productive asset, recognized and supported.

The result is that those who work in theatre in Italy often feel marginalized. Invisible. Precarious. And the question, "Yes, but what do you really do for a living?" is still very common. Even for actors. Unless you have appeared on television or in film, you are not considered a true professional. If you only do theatre, you almost don't exist.

This contributes to distancing theatre from the public. It makes it elitist, remote, and invisible. And in my opinion, this is a serious problem. Because if theatre loses its popular dimension, it loses a fundamental part of itself.

Directing and Acting: A Complicated Balance

In the best of all possible worlds, I believe that directing and acting should remain distinct roles. The director needs distance: they must be able to view the performance from the outside, to grasp the whole, to maintain clarity. The actor, on the other hand, needs to be inside: to live the scene from within, to inhabit it, to get a little lost in it. Merging these two dimensions is not impossible, but it is certainly complicated.

It has happened to me. But when it does, I always try to carve out very small, almost marginal roles for myself. And I leave the work on those scenes until the end, once the rest of the show is already built, rehearsed, and settled. This way, I can approach them first as a director—with an objective eye—and only later as an actor. But even then, I need an external eye, someone who watches me and tells me how I'm working. Because when you're on stage, you're never a reliable judge of yourself.

The director's task is to construct, harmonize, and guide. They have to hold the whole thing together. If they get too caught up in the details, if they step onto the stage, they risk losing the overall picture. And the opposite is true as well: an actor who directs themselves risks splitting their focus, constantly stepping in and out, and losing spontaneity. Often, you end up doing a half-hearted job on both fronts. And in the long run, it shows.

In some cases, I have had to replace an actor in a show I had already directed. In that situation, it's different: the structure is already there, the framework is defined, the choices have been made. It's possible to step into the role with more clarity. Even though, to be honest, there's a different risk: unconsciously imitating the actor who played the role before you. Playing not so much the character as the actor who used to play the character.

Then there are the cases where I am alone on stage. When I perform my theatrical monologues, the musical portraits—what I call *portraits*—dedicated to figures like Bob Dylan, Leonard Cohen, and BB King. In those cases, I also take care of the direction, but in a broader sense: I shape the narrative framework, the rhythm, the overall flow. It's not direction in the usual sense. It's something simpler, more essential. Storytelling theatre, relying on a different dynamic.

In those monologues, there is no fourth wall. The relationship with the audience is direct, continuous, and explicit. The staging is simpler, less elaborate. It's more a task for the actor than for the director. But it's still an interesting way to approach theatre: another channel, another form, another energy.

Even in those cases, though, I would prefer to have an external director. Someone to observe me from the outside, to help refine, shape, and polish. But often, for economic, organizational, or production reasons, that's not possible. So I rely on experience, craftsmanship, and the memory of what I have seen and learned.

I often tell younger artists: in the beginning, avoid doing both. It's not about skill, but about balance. It's hard work that requires a lot of clarity, a lot of energy. You risk constantly stepping in and out, and that can create confusion, fatigue, and uncertainty. The risk is that you lose yourself.

I do it—and continue to do it—only in very specific circumstances. When I know it's truly necessary. When I can clearly separate the two roles. But it's never my first choice.

The director is the eye. The actor is the body. Truly making them coexist, fully and deeply, is difficult. Not impossible, but rare.

Teaching Theatre, Clarifying Theatre

From the earliest years of Accademia dei Folli, we have paired our theatrical productions with a training component. We offered courses and workshops for young people and adults, starting from a simple idea: creating opportunities to approach the language of theatre through play. They were not professional training programs, but moments of theatrical literacy, of discovery. Of play, precisely.

Because theatre is also this. In many European languages, the verb used for acting is the same one used for playing: jouer, to play. In Italy, on the other hand, we often take ourselves very seriously—even when we are not doing things seriously. But I have always recognized in theatre a playful dimension, one that remains fundamental even in professional work. Every time I begin a new directing project, I invite the actors to start with play. To not have all the answers right away. To throw themselves into it with the lightness of children: "Let's pretend I was... let's pretend you were...". That's where it all begins.

Over the years, the work of directing and artistic direction has taken up more and more space, and I've drifted somewhat away from continuous teaching. But recently, I've felt the urge to return to it, choosing more specific areas. This has led to the creation of directing workshops, public speaking seminars, and intensive courses on effective communication. Sometimes aimed at schools, sometimes at professionals, sometimes at companies.

Lately, I have also had the opportunity to teach at the Holden School in Turin, alongside other writer-colleagues. In that context, I have led a module on playwriting for theatre, with a practical approach, aimed at students beginning to explore writing for the stage: training courses that are more workshop-based than theoretical, built through direct experience.

And indeed, that is precisely the aspect that interests me most: a lesson not conceived as a one-way lecture, but as a dialogue. I don't step up to a podium to deliver truths. Instead, I try to open questions, to create discussion, to offer stimulation. I believe a lesson, if it is alive, must be a space for exchange, for shared exploration. A place where we explore together. I don't have formulas, I don't have ready-made answers. I have experience to share, tools, questions. Everyone takes what they need. I am especially interested in people who are asking questions.

These training moments are precious for me too. They force you to take stock, to pause. To ask yourself why you do things a certain way. They force you to formalize, to give a name to what you normally do by instinct. And this becomes useful also in directing work, in choosing texts, in managing rehearsals. It helps you become more aware. Clearer. More effective.

My approach is always very practical. Concrete. I am interested in building something that works, that communicates. I find no gratification in building theories. I am curious to see what happens on stage, how bodies move, how words resonate.

And then there's the dialogue. Because teaching is never a one-way street. Every course is also an opportunity to learn. Every time I come home with something more. Every time my way of seeing theatre becomes clearer, richer, more renewed. That's why I always recommend, to anyone involved in theatre, to teach at least once. Even just to clarify things for themselves. Even just to see themselves from the outside. Even just to rediscover, in the eyes of others, the spark that first pushed us to begin.

The Future of Theatre (In My View)

For years, people have been saying that theatre is in crisis, that it's dying, that it can no longer keep up with the times. Personally, I don't share this view. I believe that theatre, precisely because of its nature, is one of the few art forms that cannot be replaced. No technology, however advanced, will ever be able to replicate the real encounter between a living actor and a present spectator, there in that moment.

Theatre happens in a physical place. With people. Someone speaking to someone else, at a specific time. And this thing, so simple and so concrete, has enormous value. It is a social, cultural, even political experience—in the highest and original sense of the word. It is a secular ritual. A moment in which everything stops, everything is suspended, and we are together. For an hour and a half, or two hours. All there, present. Sharing words, images, emotions, thoughts. Looking in the same direction, but each with different eyes.

It's true that today theatre no longer draws the audiences it once did. Audiences are more fragmented, and the competition from other forms of entertainment is enormous. But that doesn't mean that theatre has lost its function. On the contrary. Precisely because it is a slow, fragile, imperfect form, it has become a precious antidote. In a world that bombards us with fast, visual, digital content, theatre asks something different of us: time, attention, presence. And it offers us something that no other experience can offer with the same strength: the here and now. The uniqueness of the encounter.

In recent decades, we have seen many hybridizations: theatre and dance, theatre and video, theatre and installations, theatre and technology. These are legitimate, interesting, often fertile experiments. I too, with the Accademia dei Folli, have worked extensively on the blending of music and theatre. But I believe that, beyond all the forms, the original strength of theatre remains intact: it is presence. It is the body. It is the voice. It is one person speaking to another person. Everything else can change. That cannot.

I also love cinema, deeply. I follow it, I study it, and I live it. But cinema demands less from you. It involves you as a spectator, but it doesn't truly call you into question. Theatre does. It asks you to be there. To participate. To complete. Because unlike cinema, theatre doesn't give you everything. It gives you a trace. A sketch. And it's the spectator who finishes it, who sculpts it with their imagination, with their gaze, with their story.

On stage, we build Michelangelo's "Prisoners". It's the audience who, each night, sculpts the "Pietà". It's the audience who performs the final gesture, who transforms the whole into a completed work.

The pandemic reminded us of all this with force. When theatres remained closed for months, we felt the absence. And when they finally reopened, we also felt the hunger. The desire to return to that experience. Not out of nostalgia, but out of need. The need for real presence, for an unmediated encounter, for a living gesture.

I believe that theatre will continue to exist. That it will survive every technological revolution. But I also believe it will need to rediscover a participatory, collective vocation. It will need to return to being popular—in the noblest sense of the word. A theatre that dialogues with its audience, that listens to it, that challenges itself. A theatre that abandons self-referentiality. That does not stand on a pedestal, but sits in a circle.

This doesn't mean creating interactive shows or letting the audience decide what happens. It means recognizing that the spectator is part of the work. That without them, theatre does not exist.

And that is precisely its strength. Its beauty. The reason why, in my view, it will never die.

Perhaps it's a utopia. But it's a utopia worth continuing to seek. And I, for my part, will keep walking in that direction.

Chapter 12
Meeting Ourselves Improving Our Life Through Theatre

Mario Bois

"Io", Our Background and the Others: Going for a Walk

For all these years I have always asked myself great questions, regarding the sense of our existence, human beings and their way of life: what are the goals that we should run for. I always thought and I go on thinking that happiness is our main goal that increases the quality of life on top. We should keep in constant touch with ourselves and investigate deeper and deeper into who we are, to understand what is the best way for us and what are our personal guidelines that we can follow to reach our goals and to conquer our happiness. I guess that acting is our best friend, that allows us a sort of inner purification and strengthens the perception of ourselves. It is a way of expression that I set on three levels. First level: it involves us, our "io" (a wonderful monosyllabic word that in Italian indicates "me" the first person in conjugation but also psychological and philosophical connections), our light, our energy, but also the dark side of our moon. Second, it involves our social and cultural background, putting in evidence our setting and our perspectives about what we live in the areas of influence of our everyday actions. Third, it involves others, in a sort of continuous exchange of actions and reactions, that activates, modifies, improves and definitely changes the shading of our personality and way of being.

M. Bois (✉)
APM School, Saluzzo, Italy

Teatro del Poi, Bra, Italy
e-mail: grafica@mariobois.it

P. Corvo, I. Riccioni (eds.), *Theatre and Quality of Life*, Social Indicators Research Series 91, https://doi.org/10.1007/978-3-032-09731-6_12

We "Make" and Not Simply "Remake"

It sounds so weird when people in Italy talk about "recitare". I have grown a kind of intolerance about this verb, since it comes from the merging of "re-" (as a sort of repetition) and "citare" (that literally means "to check the list of people called to be present in a law court for a trial"). So, is that what we do? Do we merely "repeat" something? Do we really "remake" and imitate what other people do?

Are we called to be judged for what we are and what we become? Absolutely not. If I think about what this verb literally means, I immediately disagree with the "process" scene, because one of the first feelings that we should promote when we act is the one of being free and be in complete suspension of judgement. Specifically acting is a dimension in which there is no right or wrong in what we are: our body is right, our gestures and movements are right, our personality is right. No one is allowed to criticize any particular aspect, according to their individual beliefs. So we are free to be ourselves and, undoubtedly, this condition destroys all the limits that our sense of guilt, that our habit of comparison, that our fragile need for self-approval can build. And we are very experienced in building walls, limits, boundaries inside and outside ourselves. The second matter for the suspension of judgement involves our social and cultural background: we are allowed to forget all the influences that we have received from our family, our school, and all our social relationships, by the common sense and that built our perspectives. We can erase everything and draw our artwork on a white canvas. What we think and what we create on stage, what we imagine and set as true for our characters comes with dignity and is allowed to be. The third aspect is the suspension of judgement for the "others". The others are our partners on stage, the people that we meet everyday, and the characters that we welcome. In this case there is no chance of involving ethical matters for an evaluation of the others. The "others" are what they are. Our characters are what they are and they are welcomed just as they are, not affected by our personal manipulation. No need for approvals: we don't need to be approved by anyone; our social and cultural habits don't need to be approved by anyone; our characters don't need to be approved by anyone. Everything is. Everything evolves. Everything becomes. Everything is in constant transformation. In every acting process we start naked as when we were born. This is the basis of our wellness, of our joy, of our constant improvement. We start naked and all the clothes that we wear are given by "the truth": they appear at once and we believe in them. Only when we believe in what we are, "*hic et nunc*", can we involve partners and audience into our stories. How can we reach a peaceful feeling if we think of being naked? When we were born we were naked, and apart from crying for the loss of our first home (into our mother's comfortable womb), we have no filters towards other people. In case they see us naked… it is okay: we are naked! And so, what? And in those circumstances we spontaneously love playing, we laugh and play, we laugh when we play.

Let's Play!

Very far from thinking about "re-citare" as the right Italian verb to give sense to our acting process, I'd rather portray this powerful, human, expression of energy as the ability to "play". Isn't that what we normally say in other languages? In England and in the United States, as well as in all the countries that use English as their first language, "they… play", and this verb is much more concentrated or translated as interpretation (further than being the same word for ludic entertainments and for musical performances with instruments). In France and French-speaking countries acting and giving life to characters is "jouer". In Germany it is "spielen" and the actor is a "Schauspieler" who plays aspects. So why don't we play? Why don't we see ourselves or put ourselves "in a play"? That's the way: putting off our everyday clothes, getting back to being naked and playing as a child. We use to play when we are children. Then we lose this wonderful way to discover and investigate the world and the people who live in it. There could be many reasons for this paralysis of joy, creativity and artistic expression. More differently from other European countries, Italy was overwhelmed by common, widespread ways of educating people, of setting precise rules, of growing babies as adults since childhood, of running without tasting time. It was a sense of religiousness, responsibility, honour, respectability and many other convictions that always set men in chains. But I don't want to detail here a social analysis of the pillars of our culture and how these have infected our playful freedom. I want to write about playing and freeing our "io".

How I Built My Point of View

I always loved feeling my heart beating, I always loved what I am not used to call a job. As it is not simply a job. It is a way of living, a way of "playing" during all the time that we are given in our life. I always loved playing. I always loved life. I have fed my curiosity since childhood, everything has affected my senses and sensibility. So I started learning and I have been going on learning for over 40 years. This gave me and gives me the chance to understand that what I have already learnt is in constant transformation, that life is in constant transformation through the experiences that change our ways of feeling our existence and its relationship with other people and with the different backgrounds in which we set ourselves. I had many guiding lights, who enlightened my joy and filled my lungs with deep, pure air, coming from supreme arts, from the pure desire of being, becoming, and expressing. My flight to remember and think of them is starred with genuine endless thanks. They positively changed me, provoked me to act and to react, and made me feel that being "one", "true" and "individual" was my first responsibility in respect of myself and of all the people around me. I started to love deeper. I started to love myself deeper. And then I started to love sharing.

Energy, Enthusiasm and Sharing

Three words are pillars for me to build a connection with playing, with acting: energy, enthusiasm and sharing. Energy is the lifeblood, it is our five senses in action, it is every morning when we wake up, it is our curiosity for a deep perception of ourselves, of others and of the world. It is our sunlight that really makes us feel like a star. Enthusiasm is the gasoline to develop energy, it is the consciousness of rightness, it is the way of feeding experiences pervaded by our energy. Sharing is "me" among "the others", it is the building of connections, it is the epiphany of the personal meaning that we give to a performance, when this is not just a way of satisfying our "ego" but the extension of our powerful feelings in a dimension of constant evolution and comparison that erase every bad feeling of competition with the strength of "being", "doing" and "growing" together.

A Horizontal Relationship

When people asked me to "teach" this was another verb that left me stuck in emptiness. What a presumption it would be to call me "teacher", to assign myself the role of a leader, to charge myself with the responsibility expected by other people trusting in my secret power and endless knowledge. No, not me. I am a "sharer", an "energy dispenser", "an enlighter of epiphanies". The relationship that grows between a guide and all the people in a group should always be a horizontal one, made of mutual confidence, made of mutual respect, made of mutual awareness of the richness that every human being holds, can express and can enhance when not left alone. I don't mean of forgetting roles, as one is the guide and should be strongly responsible and aware of this, but it's fundamental that this role doesn't put a boundary, doesn't overwhelm the generous necessity of creating a flow of sharing.

Let Our Brains Sleep, Create and Act!

And so, here I am. Always learning, every "today", how to deal with people (perhaps) a little better than "yesterday". And, besides this, I try to be constantly in empathy and connected with the potential power of growing up and improving individual self-consciousness. But we don't come to paint, with the evidence of a white canvas in front of us. As written before, we have luggage full of experiences that we carry with us and that can be really helpful for living characters and situations on stage. Nevertheless, every creation can be purer if it comes from a white surface, from the temporary forgetfulness of our "comfort zone" and of our personal habits. In this way we feed our opportunity to grow up and to discover the dark side of our moon. Everybody is a wonderful diamond crossed by different fades of lights: once some colours come out, sometimes others, sometimes some colours are refused by ourselves, since they don't belong to our ordinary behaviour.

That's the starting point: let's erase the traces on the canvas, let's close the books opened until this present moment and, for a while, let's be "in suspension of disbelief" (as William Wordsworth suggested), excited by the chance of creating something new and free to assign the role of creators to our impulse and feeling, rather than our rationality. We can partially switch the logic side of our brain off. We can give power to our body and to cellular memory, to the evolution of sensations into perceptions and then feelings. To the discovery of the endless variety of "possible ourselves". The question is: if we refer to "possible ourselves" how can I transfer these identities to characters? Don't they remain in my ordinary area of action, in my everyday life, even if they get different facets? This belongs to a second phase of our creation: the chance of mirroring our personal experiences and our deepest discoveries in our characters' life.

Our characters walk (as we can walk), breathe (as we can breathe), eat, drink, smile, cry, shout (as we are able to do all these things). But the cocktail we make is the result of crossing our personal experiences and feelings with the given circumstances of the biography of a character. To give birth to these new identities we can even take inspiration from other people that we meet every day and, through a patient and precise observation, make all these habits, feeling, and ways of living ours, not imitating them but really feeling them. That is the cocktail: the selected faces of the multiple "ourselves" shaken and merged with the selected details that we can empirically get by external inferences.

Awareness: Forget the Limits and Welcome the New!

But I don't want to look like a teacher, in these few lines. Much more I'd like to be an observer, astonished by the multiple chances that come out from training ourselves to act. This white canvas is for everyone the consciousness of being totally free. We can cut the chains that tie us to the past, to everything that was built either by others or by the context. And we can start to write a new story. In this sense our "quality of life" becomes one of the main goals. Freedom is the centre of the improvement of our quality of life, but it's not just a rhetorical thought. Abandoning all the boundaries, the locks, the rules, we can feel free in different ways. Free to discover. Free to laugh. Free to know. Free to understand. Free to forget. Free to fail! Mistakes, failures, and fear of external judgements lead us to suffer from these conditions. That makes sense: when we cut the chains all this discomfort vanishes.

But this is just a first benefit. The second benefit comes out thanks to the opportunity to discover: erasing our comfort zone, we think about our "*io*" as a new land to conquer, thus giving any feature as possible, any feeling as liveable, any action as feasible. There are no limits. And we welcome the new. For example: you can be a quiet person, never crossed, never angry. One day, during your training and your painting on your white canvas you discover a shout, a rough movement of your arm, a bad glance…

You could say that anger is not healthy, and of course this can be a nice point of view. But this is just the possible expression of anger and it is a virtual situation in which you can express it. So the steps are: to live the feeling, to become completely aware of it (collecting and analysing all the physical and emotional details), to think that this new feeling could belong to us (even if it's not part of our daily behaviour), to be free to use it on stage as a natural way of our expression. Objection: does this process transform us into someone else? Maybe, or maybe better we can say that it unveils us and our deepest and darkest sides. Second objection: does this process alter our daily behaviour? It can, but only if we let it do it so: when we are out of the stage, we must recognize our identity and personality. We can think of becoming much more experienced, much more skilled. We can think about all our discoveries, but, in other words, we encourage changes in our identity and personality, only if this makes us happy.

And here we touch the third benefit: happiness. As written before, I think that happiness should be for everybody the main target of our life. Life is mainly a beautiful, individual experience driven by our "io". Then our "io" meets other people. But, first of all, it is individual: it involves our personality in acting and reacting. I always tease during training or acting sessions, saying: "They say I am mortal, but until I don't prove it '*hic et nunc*', nobody, except for me, will know if and when I will die". It's a joke to underline the personal point of view and the personal way that is up to each one's life. So happiness should be a common aim for everybody. If we consider this—the pursuit of happiness—as a possible way of life, we can explore how we can be happy by freeing ourselves from chains, by becoming aware of our revealed potentialities and by leading ourselves and by allowing ourselves to make them come true. Under this light, happiness becomes the chance of independent and free governance of ourselves.

We can act/react, driven by a specific emotion, but in the centre of our body this feeling can (or not) come out and become visible for others. I will try to explain better. Let's go back to rage. Every feeling is caused by something: facts, interactions, previous evolving feelings. We can really feel anger, due to an unpleasant event or to a strong argument. In that case we cannot say that we are happy. But happiness lives in the chance of managing the anger and choosing if and how to express it. It is a fact much more of instinct and impulse, rather than rationality, but our brain helps us to balance everything. And that's why we can be happy by reaching a personal spontaneous self-control or better self-management: it is not a chain, it is a constantly increasing awareness. We feel able and free to act and react. We don't feel led by anyone else. And that's why we feel happier and our quality of life improves.

How Art Can Help

This is my general thought about the process. But improving our life is a matter of someway solving our problems, overcoming diseases, embarrassments… Art can help. Art comes to help. In many cases I have seen the power of art in turning on the light over dark dead ends. People who have difficulties with fluent speech. People who have difficulties with the outcome of their personal thoughts or feelings. People who have difficulties with shyness, physical contact or quiet relationships with others. People who have disabilities. All these are pictures of the precise moment when they come and decide to start the trip, this personal wonderful trip that will lead them to take a look at themselves from an external point, that will allow them to dress new clothes… And, little by little, step by step, if they don't fear welcoming opportunities, all this happens.

Respect Yourself and Your Rhythms

It is an evolution that I have noticed with no particular difference due to age. It happens with children. It even happens with adolescents. But it even happens with adult people. Of course, the more a man is locked, the longer it will be for him or her to free themselves from constrictions. Usually children (but it is not a rule) have to struggle with a shorter period of life, in which their personal luggage has been influenced by family, schools and some other places. Adult people are much more inserted into the world: that means that their relationships have built solid convictions, walls, rules, comfort habits, prejudices… So we can say in a simple way that being younger helps to make it faster to clean our canvas and start to paint. But it's not always like this. Anyway we are not a factory of happiness that needs to be much more productive and needs to accelerate processes. Of course the sooner we have results, the sooner we can feel free and better. But we need to allow our body and mind to follow our steps and our personal way to trace this process. And that's a respectful condition, that further increases our "quality of life". It is our rhythm, our time, we choose it, minute by minute: we can accelerate or slow down and it's always right. For us. As it must be right just for us. For our personal experience of improvement. Becoming more aware of ourselves, of our potentiality, we strengthen a condition that is the most important signal for freedom and happiness: respect. We need to respect our "io", to respect our rhythm, our way of thinking, our needs, our way of looking at the world and at other people. And we expect respect from others that are welcome to meet our uniqueness, but gently, gradually, consciously, in a word respectfully.

The Energy of the Group

I have been conducting classes, workshops and periodical dates with groups of people and I would like to spend some words telling how the energy of a group can help individuality and individual goals. Every group is a magical mix of lives, experiences, personalities and points of view. Every group acts and reacts to each participant and to each input in a different way. That's why it is important, as we do in our life, to keep a perfect balance and to manage individualities as a part of the group. Nobody should feel superior or inferior to other people: everyone is like a ring of a necklace and balance is the neck that shows all of us as precious jewels. In the group, contrasts meet, different points of view evolve and the constant exercise of working with music, movements and involvement of our body gives new shapes to our sculpture. We become alternately sculptors and sculptures, leading the game with a complete freedom of creativity or being led to feel ourselves as an artwork. In both cases we are deeply part of a process that helps us feel all the shades of the truth. Specifically, in groups that include people with disabilities, I really have to say that the exchange of resources empower all the members of the group, helping to destruct limits that for each person were built differently—as said before—or caused differently. People help each other through the power of theatre, of acting, of being, of feeling.

"Building": A Concrete Sample

Recent format that I created is called "Building" and concerns the opportunity for each participant in a group to create his/her own character, walking along two main ways: personal preferences and real life. I asked each member of the group of thinking about characters that they like (in literature, cinema, theatre) following their personal preferences. Second step: I asked them to think about a man or woman that they usually meet during everyday life (excluding direct relatives and best friends). Third, I asked them to feel deeply in connection with the two characters that they had chosen and to let them live together inside themselves, selecting and merging their features. People have complete freedom to create their new character, but according to precise given circumstances (the ones that come out from the story of their "famous" character) and chosen habits (the ones that they experience, exploring the "real" world of the character they meet every day). That's why I wanted to call this experience "Building", which actually has two meanings: one regarding the creation of the characters and the second regarding the coincidence by which all the characters live in the same building. I set three different rooms: one for cutting the ropes with our comfort zone and our everyday habits, the second for meeting the character and feeling the *hic et nunc* with him/her while starting to paint on a white canvas and the third that involves the set and that can have two different roles. It can be the "Garden", a place of the "Building" where all the characters meet and can experience relationships with others. It can be strictly "Building" when it becomes alternately the house of each character in which they live their daily life. At the end of our work in the "Building" a long time is dedicated to leaving the character and getting back to our ordinary life. This way of taking distance from our common role, from our comfort zone, allows us to discover new chances, not imitating, but making them possibilities of our own. We are allowed to go far from ourselves and to explore something unusual, but that somehow we start to like. We own new instruments not only to create, but also to face what happens every day. Not only on stage but also in our real life. This makes us stronger, smarter and more confident.

Back Home

Back to an improved life. In conclusion I can say that the importance of joining and practicing activities such as physical training, physical theatre, acting, sensorial memory, and emotional memory, leads to results both in the disciplines we face and in our lives. When we get back home, when we get back to what we consider our real everyday life we have enriched our luggage and we have put some new clothes in it and, above all, the knowledge of how to dress them. We have some more magic to live everyday as a new special day and, I do believe, to improve our way of dreaming and to make our dreams come true.

Acknowledgements Growing up as an artist is a hard process: my thankful and special thoughts go to Nuccio Cantamutto, Valter Scarafia, Elide Giordanengo, Danny Lemmo, Sergei and Gennadi Ostrenko, and Mamadou Dioume. Supporting an artist, sharing his unbalanced life and agreeing with his dreams is the hardest thing: a special thanks goes to my parents, Laura and Ettore, and to my partner Valentina. A special further thanks to Paolo Corvo for his invitation to write and to my friend Beppe Incarbona, with whom I share the love for art and acting: he has been allowing me to improve projects, workshops and ideas.

GPSR Compliance

The European Union's (EU) General Product Safety Regulation (GPSR) is a set of rules that requires consumer products to be safe and our obligations to ensure this.

If you have any concerns about our products, you can contact us on

ProductSafety@springernature.com

In case Publisher is established outside the EU, the EU authorized representative is:

Springer Nature Customer Service Center GmbH
Europaplatz 3
69115 Heidelberg, Germany

www.ingramcontent.com/pod-product-compliance
Lightning Source LLC
Chambersburg PA
CBHW060320260626
47214CB00048B/12
9783032097309